Fat Wars

Fat Wars

45 Days to Transform Your Body

Brad J. King

MACMILLAN CANADA
TORONTO

First published in Canada in 2000 by
Macmillan Canada, an imprint of CDG Books Canada

Canadian Cataloguing in Publication Data

King, Brad (Brad J.)
     Fat wars : 45 ways to transform your body

Includes index.
ISBN 0-7715-7692-7

1. Weight loss. 2. Reducing diets. I. Title.

RM222.2.K56 2000   613.2'5   C00-931435-0

Cover photo by David Hanover/Stone
Author photo by Scope Photography, Victoria, B.C.
Cover design by CS Richardson
Text design and typesetting by Kim Monteforte/Heidy Lawrance Associates

Macmillan Canada
An imprint of CDG Books Canada Inc.
Toronto

Printed in Canada

     5 6 TRANS 04 03 02 01

Contents

FOREWORD

As a nutritional researcher with a traditional background, I have spent many years watching the successes and failures of traditional medical practices on weight loss.

The scientific approach is the right one, but researchers, authors and health professionals must keep open minds, look at all the evidence and be willing to change their assumptions when findings don't support them.

In this inspiring book, Brad King has compiled conclusive evidence on the benefits of adopting a new lifestyle that incorporates a dietary strategy and a sustainable exercise protocol to let you—once and for all—lose weight intelligently. Brad's approach is scientifically grounded with a refreshing and comfortable approach that guides you step-by-step-by-step. Ancient wisdom and modern science coalesce into an easy-to-follow prescription that works. Yes, it really works!

You hold in your hands a remarkably helpful book. It will explain why many of us may be fat in the first place. It is chock-full of tips on how to incorporate proven exercise strategies and healthy eating habits into your day-to-day life that will, at long last, result in permanent fat reduction. It is the information you need to help you navigate through a sometimes confusing world where weight-loss misinformation is the rule rather than the exception.

As important as the material in this "must read" book is, it is the enthusiasm and commitment of its researcher and writer that strikes you deeply. Brad takes your hand and leads you through the land mines of confusion toward a dietary and exercise strategy that allows you to eat abundantly while spending less time exercising and lose critical pounds quickly. You may have heard this claim before. However, this book is different from any other because it approaches weight loss from a new perspective, the one that proves that not all weight is bad. *Fat Wars* is a triumph. You will not only finally be able to shed those excess pounds, but also it is likely that your life will be extended, overall health improved, energy and endurance boosted, appetite controlled and your concepts about food and exercise radically changed for the better. A healthy diet and an exercise program are the cornerstones of a healthy lifestyle. Good food should provide pleasure and satisfaction as well as nourishment, and should support rather than undermine the body's natural healing potential. Exercise should be gratifying rather than confusing.

Look beyond the failures of your past and follow the steps as Brad guides you through. You will be thrilled by the positive results. I find this book fascinating and genuine—it adds an exciting new dimension to the real secrets of permanent fat loss.

Bravo to you, Brad King, for your diligent research and sincere dedication! Bravo to you, the reader—it is as simple as becoming aware of how you became overweight to begin with, and then taking the necessary steps to gain victory, one battle at a time. You will never regret it. The time to begin is now! Bon appétit.

I wish you abundant good health.

Sam Graci
Author, *The Power of Superfoods*
Researcher and Formulator of GREENS+

ACKNOWLEDGEMENTS

It has always been my dream to write a book on fat loss. After my many lectures on the topic, I have always been approached by people who were asking for one. There was just too much information to digest in an hour-and-a-half talk. It is for these people, as well as others, who are both confused and frustrated by the propaganda of the diet industry that I thank for the creation of *Fat Wars*.

There are many people who have encouraged me to write this book. Without the support and selflessness of these people, this book may not have come to fruition. I wish to pay a special thanks to the following people who have played a role in one way or another to the success of this project.

First thanks to my soul mom, Peggy Groom, who not only adopted me when my own mother passed away, but who has supported me and pushed me to complete the project; I love you with all my heart, Peggy. I am grateful to one of my mentors, Sam Graci, whose commitment to helping anyone who was smart enough to listen has inspired me to be the researcher, lecturer and health advocate I am today. Thanks to another mentor, Dr. Michael Schmidt, who has always supported me and whom I have come to admire in both business and friendship. Also thanks go to Dr. Kenneth Seaton, from whom I have learned so much. A special thanks to Stewart Brown, for believing enough in my work to support this project. Thanks to one of my greatest supporters of all, Fred Hagadorn, who has not only believed in me since the beginning but has continually put his name on the line to make sure others did as well. Thank you, Deane Parkes, for giving me the chance to show my stuff when I was just starting out. Thanks to my editor, Susan Girvan, for putting up with my perfectionism on the project and still keeping it layman friendly. Thanks to Robert Harris, publisher of CDG Books Canada, for getting pumped about the idea and putting your company's name behind it. Thanks to everyone at Greens+ (ehn Inc.) for their continued enthusiasm and support. A special thanks to Tara Stubensey, for not only reading over the manuscript, but actually getting excited about it. Thanks to David Chapman and the Purity Life group, where I first got a taste of what the health industry is all about. Thank you to Linda Lewis for being a business partner and a friend and helping me balance three years of radio life with three years of lecturing on the road. Thanks to Terry Spence and the CFAX 1070 group for giving me my start in radio. Thanks to my good friend and supporter Naomi Kolesnikff, who has been there for me from the beginning. Thank you to fellow researcher, Rick Brunner, Ph.D., for helping me with some of the research for the book. A warm thanks and love to my three sisters, Debbie, Lisa (you will always be my little sister) and Chris.

Special thanks go out to all the researchers of the world who tirelessly search for new ways to battle the bulge and end the Fat Wars once and for all.

—Brad J. King
September 2000

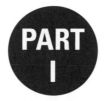

So We're Fat.
So What?

North Americans are getting progressively fatter every day. In the U.S., over one half of men and women over the age of 20 are considered over-fat; in Canada, it's almost one-third. Obesity rates are also soaring. Between 1978 and 1992 rates of obesity in Canada went from 6.8% to 12% in men, and 9.6% to 14% in women. The problem is not just in North America. In countries like Western Samoa, 58% of adult men and 76% of adult women are obese.

Our ideal weight is the weight at which our risk of dying prematurely is statistically the lowest. "Obese" is usually defined as 20% or more above our ideal weight. Over-fat is somewhat less fat than that. Establishing an ideal (and actual) weight can be an exact science. However, most of us use something less precise that takes into account our height, our bone structure (fine or heavy) and how much muscle we have on our frames. Generally speaking, we know when we're carrying too much body fat. So, is this just a matter of us wearing bigger clothes? Is it just about looking bad and feeling worse? Isn't this a personal choice?

Yes and no. Being over-fat goes in and out of fashion, but it also sets us up for a whole host of ailments such as heart disease, diabetes, high cholesterol, high blood pressure, stroke, cancers (gastrointestinal, prostate, breast, endometrial, etc.), plus gallbladder disease, immune dysfunction, gallstones, sleep apnea, infertility, lower back pain and arthritis. The fatter we are, the greater our chances of suffering from one or more of these.

Cardiovascular disease comes early when we're over-fat because the blood vessels in our legs, or the microcapillaries in our eyes (to name but two) simply begin to wear out faster. They can actually fail three times as quickly as they do in someone who is lean. Too much body fat also greatly increases the risk of developing high blood pressure.

Being over-fat plays a huge role in the development of Type 2 diabetes. This used to be strictly an adult disease, but today, the marked increase in over-fat children is mirrored by a similar increase in childhood Type 2 diabetes. (Kids are also suffering more from asthma and depression—remember how cruel kids can be at times?—because they're over-fat.) There are about 18 million people with Type 2 diabetes in North America, about half of them undiagnosed. By dropping excess body fat, 15 million would likely take less medication, have more energy, greatly improve their health and live longer. Of those with diabetes, it's estimated that 85% are over-fat; many are obese. Their condition sets them up for a host of diabetes-related complications, including blindness, kidney failure, heart disease and amputations.

Cancer too? Over 70% of all cancers are attributed to lifestyle. When we factor out those cancers related to smoking tobacco and drinking alcohol, many of the rest are linked with being over-fat. These cancers are instigated by estrogens and carcinogens—stored in our fat cells. This is where they find a home; if they don't have a place to stay, they can't do the damage.

And, of course, if our immune systems are constantly doing battle with estrogens, carcinogens, etc., they become overworked. According to Dr. Edward Conley, the medical director of the Fatigue and Fibromyalgia Clinic of Michigan, "The immune system has to kill about 200 cancers a day, and if our immune system is strong, it kills 200 a day." Don't forget— our immune systems are not only working to keep cells from mutating into cancer, they are also dealing with numerous other organisms like viruses, parasites and bacterial infections. Studies also show that obesity places undue strain on an already compromised situation by decreasing the body's ability to deal with stress.

In addition, many researchers believe that it's not just how fat we are that affects our risk of disease, but where the fat is stored. Recent research has shown that body fat in the stomach area, as opposed to body fat on the thighs and butt, is one of the main causes of disease. This gut fat is related to an excessive production of hormones that surge into the bloodstream during stress and reduce our immunity. The more belly fat we have, the higher the risk of premature death. In addition, tummy fat cells seem to be especially good at dumping lipids (fats) into the bloodstream, which is not good either.

This is more than just a cosmetic issue: it's also a serious health issue, with these diseases quietly costing all of us billions of dollars each year. The direct cost of obesity in Canada has been estimated to be 2.4% of the health care budget, with the three largest money sinkholes being high blood pressure, diabetes and heart disease. In the U.S., obesity is estimated to account for 5.7% of the national health expenditure—over $100 billion per year. There's also an indirect financial cost related to lost productivity due to health-related absenteeism.

Too Short for Your Weight?

Is there such a thing as an ideal weight range? Yes! How do we find out what that is? Researchers who study the effects of body fat on health often refer to a person's Body Mass Index or BMI. This is a number they calculate by using a formula that takes into account both weight and height. (Yes, size matters.) This BMI rating has become a common way to quickly judge whether your weight is putting you in a high-risk health category. How do they know this? A lot of research has been done. For example, a study published in 1995 by Manson and colleagues followed the health of 115,000 nurses for 14 to 16 years. The lowest mortality rate was found in women with a BMI of 19 or less. The risk of premature death increased by 20% for those with BMIs in the 19 to 24.9 range, 60% for BMIs of 27 to 28.9, and double the risk of premature death for those with a BMI of 29 and higher.

The ideal BMI is considered to be between 19 and 25. (The average BMI of a female in the U.S. is 26.) You can figure out your own BMI through a simple series of calculations that start by dividing your weight in pounds by your height in feet squared. Then multiply this figure by 4.89. It sounds like something only a mathematician could do, but it's really not that hard.

Here's an example. A person who weighs 125 lbs. and stands 5 feet, 3 inches tall (5.25 feet) would divide 125 by 27.5625 (5.25 × 5.25). The result is 4.535, which is then multiplied by 4.89 to give a BMI rating of 22.2. This is in the healthy range. If that same person weighed 150 lbs., the BMI rating would be 150, divided by 27.5625. The resulting 5.442 would then be multiplied by 4.89 for a BMI of 26.6 Time to do something!

There is one caution with this standard: A lean, heavily muscled person will likely have a BMI rating that puts them in the danger zone, when in fact they are healthy. Don't forget: the body is comprised of lean body mass (tissue, bone and muscle) which weighs significantly more than fat does. For example, I personally weigh 190 pounds and stand 5 feet, 8 inches tall (5.67 feet). If I divide 190 by 32.1489 (5.67 squared), and then multiply the result by 4.89, I come up with a body mass index of 29.

In this particular scenario, the BMI would be wrong. (Of course it would be!) You see, I am actually in good shape. (No really, I am). The true measure of obesity is the percentage of overall fat on the body. A normal healthy man should not exceed a body fat percentage of 15, while the healthy limit for a woman is between 15% and 22%. I carry a body fat percentage at the moment of 13. This is about the amount of fat a male athlete carries, and since I am an athlete of sorts, this makes sense.

As you begin to win your personal Fat War, you will be building muscle. For most, this will not result in a high BMI rating, and the BMI will remain a useful measure. Nevertheless, it is highly advisable for anyone interested in their true health to get their overall fat composition measured. See Appendix I for recommendations on how to get this done.

The theory of premature mortality is no vague threat. Most over-fat and obese people are likely to check out before their time. Given the list of diseases noted earlier, it's not surprising that those of us who fall into that category rarely reach the ripe old age of 80 or 90. (In Western Samoa, life expectancy is 67 years for men and not quite 72 for women. Think that's long enough?) The social cost of premature deaths mustn't be overlooked. Not only have we lost people who could have made major contributions to society for many years to come, but people who were grandmothers and grandfathers, aunts and uncles, and moms and dads to people who loved them and whom they loved, are all gone—thanks to fat. Being over-fat does not automatically doom us to illness and premature death, but it certainly increases our risk of being one of the statistics.

Fat Wars is about helping to decrease the risk of premature death by moving ourselves into a healthy weight range. It's about understanding how the body works, and working with what nature designed. We can speed up metabolism, burn stored body fat, increase our ability to fight disease, create more energy and just plain feel better. Anyone who's tried to lose fat knows it's a tough battle. The news in *Fat Wars* is that what you don't know will make you lose the fight. *Fat Wars* will show you how to transform your body, and make yourself the victor.

1

The Skinny on Fat—
The Generator and The Furnace

Why is it that some people can eat and eat and eat, and never seem to gain a pound, while the rest of us gain weight by just looking at food? *Why* is it that when a woman and a man go on the same diet (and stick to it), he seems to lose the weight faster than she does? What makes the difference? The efficiency of two body processes: metabolism, which many of us are vaguely familiar with, and its subordinate, thermogenesis, which may be something new to you.

Metabolism is the series of biochemical reactions that takes place inside our cells (all 100 trillion of them!) to create energy. Our bodies take the basic fuel components that we give them (carbohydrates, dietary fats and dietary proteins, aka food) and break them down to produce the energy we use to keep warm, move muscles, breathe, blink—it's the force that keeps the machinery functioning. Our bodies either use this fuel on the spot or (you knew this was coming) store it in our bodies' fat cells for later use. Of the energy that's used on the spot, approximately 80% is released as heat, while the rest does the other work. A fast, efficient metabolism can produce a lot of energy and heat (and consume a lot of fuel).

Thermogenesis is a slightly different body cell process: this time, stored energy (body fat) is burned just to produce heat. Again, the efficiency of our thermogenic systems can mean the difference between average or over-abundant fat stores.

In short, each of our bodies has a generator and a furnace.

THE GENERATOR

Most people think our digestive systems break down our food and use it directly as energy. They don't. We first have to convert the carbo-hydrates, dietary fats and dietary proteins into a universal energy sub-stance; scientists call it adenosine triphosphate or ATP. Each one of our cells has a tiny biochemical factory that can produce ATP, an organic compound that is stored in muscle tissue. When the brain sends a signal along the nervous system to trigger a muscle contraction, enzymes break down ATP to release the energy required for the job. All our energy starts with ATP. It's depleted rapidly, and, as you can guess, there are so many require-ments to move muscles (pump a heart, scratch a head, click a remote, move a piano) that although ATP is constantly being made, it's also constantly being used up. It's the required basic fuel for energy that doesn't require oxygen (short term) and for energy that does (longer term, aerobic efforts).

While ATP is the basic element of human energy, our amazing bodies have a complex and wonderful system to keep us moving in a variety of ways. In essence, we have different levels in our energy system, depending on the type of physical activity involved and how much oxygen we need at the time. Think of it as working the way we change gears in a car.

First Gear: ATP

For immediate energy, we can get along just by using ATP. Our bodies make this constantly, but it's not stored as pure ATP in large quantities. ATP alone can power our muscles when we throw a ball or swing a tennis racquet—efforts that last for about three seconds.

Second Gear: ATP, CP

For a more sustained effort, the muscles pull in a second fuel compo-nent: creatine phosphate or CP. This is an energy source that can be stored longer than ATP and is available to juice up the fuel mix when ATP runs out. What's really happening is that CP donates its phosphate atom to what's left after ATP is broken down and, *voila*, we have more ATP to keep us going for up to 10 seconds. During this time we can do a sprint or wrestle a pair of shoes onto a small child.

Third Gear: ATP, CP, Glucose ... and Lactic Acid

If we need energy for more than 10 seconds—say for up to two minutes—we go into third gear. At this point, the muscles are using ATP and calling on CP to help make more quick fuel. In addition, glucose and glycogen are being broken down to help turn more spent ATP into usable fuel.

A by-product of the glucose breakdown is lactic acid. Hydrogen ions released from excess lactic acid makes our muscles burn—a clear signal for us to either stop what we're doing because we don't have the fuel to take us any further in this effort, or add oxygen to the fuel mix. Time to take a deep breath and go to the next level.

Fourth Gear: Oxygen Overdrive (the Aerobic Phase)

If the energy needs are for longer than two minutes, we must add oxygen to the fuel mix in order to carry on. Let's face it—most of the things we do last longer than two minutes. This is where conditioning comes in: we all know that oxygen utilization is a key indicator of fitness. That's because the more efficiently our bodies can use oxygen, the longer we're able to generate enough energy for long-term, strenuous effort.

At this stage, we're still making ATP, but another part of the muscle cell (the mitochondrion) kicks in to produce long-term energy. It combines a number of elements, including oxygen and fatty acids (YES!), which burn nicely when combined with the oxygen and all the rest, to produce a sustained source of energy for activity. This is the gear that burns fat—it's like putting the car on cruise control.

Our bodies switch gears effortlessly, but aerobic gear is where we want our muscles to be in order to burn fat instead of storing it. For that, we need to do what we can to make sure our metabolism works efficiently.

THE FURNACE

While our metabolism provides both heat and energy so we can go about our daily tasks, thermogenesis just provides heat. Why do we have this auxiliary system? We are warm-blooded creatures, meant to keep our body temperatures at a constant level—98.6°F—in a changing environment. In our Canadian climate, we're usually trying to keep warm; in hot climates, the body's working hard to stay cool. Whether we're heating or cooling our surrounding environment, it takes energy to do it; the same is true of our bodies' efforts to regulate our own temperature. This is a very big job, and regardless of whether or not we need energy to do work, we always need to produce heat.

In general, heat is produced in three ways:
- through physical activity, during which the muscles create heat as they do work, enabling them to do double duty efficiently (metabolism)
- through diet-induced activity, especially when we've had a large meal that requires our digestive systems to go into overdrive (metabolism). (Do you ever notice how hot it gets after Christmas dinner?)
- through temperature regulation, when our skeletal muscle cells shiver to warm up our bodies (thermogenesis)

What Is Thermogenesis?

Thermogenesis is the chemical production of heat within the body to promote the oxidation of body fat. In order for your body to maintain a temperature of 98.6°F, it must constantly burn fat. Whenever you increase your metabolic rate, you create more heat and burn more fat. In the body, "brown fat" specializes in the burning of "white fat" (blubber). Noradrenaline is a hormone produced by the adrenal glands, which activate thermogenesis in the brown fat and muscles.

Basically, your body does three things with consumed calories: (1) it uses them to meet its daily energy needs; (2) it stores them for future energy requirements; or (3) it wastes or burns calories in special cells in the body known as brown adipose tissue (BAT). The function of the BAT cells is to burn the calories your body doesn't need. This process, called thermogenesis, means the generation of heat. Fat buildup occurs primarily when the BAT cells are not working properly or not being activated often enough. The body deals with the excess calories by storing them as body fat.

It is theorized that the sudden weight gain experienced by many between the ages of 30 to 40 may be the result of a shutdown of the BAT cell thermogenic mechanism under the influence of some genetic cue. When that happens, we must find ways to reactivate BAT cell thermogenesis and reverse the genetic trigger, or we will continue to store body fat no matter which diet we try. Fortunately, studies show that it is possible to reverse the genetic fault that makes thousands of people overweight. The process starts by mobilizing stored body fat, carrying it through the blood to the BAT cells where it is incinerated. The body converts stored body fat back into calories through thermal combustion—themogenesis. Over time, regular thermogenic activation generates the production of additional BAT cells, resulting in a dramatic increase in the calories burned as heat.

Thermogenesis helps keep us warm even when we don't require muscular energy: it's what keeps animals warm during hibernation and newborn babies warm before their metabolic systems have developed (or us, when we're sleeping). Think of thermogenesis as a metabolic helper.

How the Furnace Works

Our personal heating systems use three specialized chemical proteins, called "uncoupling proteins," to create the heat that helps to keep us warm. Our sources of these three chemical proteins are brown adipose tissue (BAT), muscle tissue, immune cells, white body fat and skeletal muscles; they are found throughout the body. These chemical proteins are called "uncoupling proteins" because the proteins used when generating energy create both heat and energy; the uncoupling proteins can separate the work of producing heat from energy production and make only heat.

Thermogenesis relies on the most abundant and economical source of fuel it can find to produce the heat: body fat. We need the body fat that we are at war with to help keep our temperatures running at 98.6°F in the shade. This is why we need some body fat in storage. The problem is that the majority of us have enough fuel stored to heat a medium-sized crowd, rather than just ourselves.

The heating process starts by mobilizing stored body fat and carrying it through the blood into the cells where the uncoupling proteins convert it to soluble fat so it can be incinerated. Over time, regular thermogenic activity can also produce additional BAT cells to increase the whole fat-burning process. As the body becomes more efficient at moving the fat through the system (that is, the BAT cells in particular are working effectively), body fat is kept to a minimum.

In keeping with our furnace analogy, we also have a thermostat. Ours is better known as the thyroid and is a major player in both the thermogenic and metabolic processes. This gland, located at the front of the neck, produces three different thyroid hormones that regulate both processes.

Aging BATs

While BAT cells can act as both generators and furnaces, and despite the many other sites for the uncoupling proteins, it's the BAT cells that are the major site for our (fat burning) thermogenesis.

As we noted, when our BAT cell processes are working at peak efficiency, body fat is at a minimum. It's been suggested that in our days of youth, when our uncoupling proteins are working at their best, BAT cells serve two functions. They prevent dietary fats from being stored as body fat by turning excess calories into waste, which can be eliminated; they also constantly convert body fat into soluble fat that can be burned up. Over time, this system becomes less efficient. Why? We start giving it less than ideal fuel, we give our systems too much fuel, our ability to produce uncoupling proteins diminishes or the process stops altogether. The sudden weight gain experienced by many of us between the ages of 30 and 40 may be the result of a dysfunction in, or a shutdown of, the thermogenic system. While BAT cells aren't the only site for fat burning, every bit helps. We have to find ways to reactivate the process. If we don't, it won't matter what diet scheme we try. We will never burn off that fat.

FIRING UP THE FAT BURNERS

Since muscle—the generator—is a prime site for fat burning, one way to get the fat burners working better is by moving those muscles through exercise. In addition, a high-protein diet has been proven to increase thermogenic activity. A 1993 study by Dr. Barenys and his colleagues at Universitat Rovira i Virgili, Reus, Spain, found that a combination of a higher-protein diet and moderate exercise increases the body's metabolic activity much more than a high-protein diet alone (or exercise alone). It was so effective that it raised the resting metabolic rate of the participants well into the day following the exercise. The reason for this metabolic enhancement may lie in dietary proteins' ability to increase the metabolic rate: a protein meal can increase that rate by 25 to 30%, compared to an increase of 4% after a carbohydrate meal.

Can we go further to find ways to crank up the furnace? Research has shown that BAT cells can be increased in humans who are exposed to cold temperatures for long periods of time (such as those living in the Arctic). If this seems like too drastic a step to take in order to burn fat, science has also isolated an ally called *Citrus aurantium* (or Bitter Orange, *zhi shi*), which is a South Asian fruit that resembles a small orange. It contains five key alkaloids that increase the breakdown of stored fat and increase the metabolic rate through thermogenesis. It shows great promise in the efforts to stimulate the fat-burning process. (More on this important nutrient in Chapter 12.)

FUEL STORAGE

Of our 100 trillion cells, around 30 billion of them can store fat. These fat cells can expand, and if that isn't enough, they can also divide to many times their natural size (in fact, up to 1,000 times). They can also shrink, but even if they shrink, they're with you for life. (The only way to make them disappear is through liposuction.) This system evolved over long centuries, back in the days when the nearest mini-mart was several thousand years away. Then we were foraging for nuts and berries, and had an occasional wild game meal. When food was plentiful, we feasted because food storage was rarely possible in those days, and it could be some time before we had lots to eat again. To get us through the feast-and-famine cycle, the human body developed the ability to convert almost anything into fat (stored fuel)—we don't have to eat fat to manufacture it. Excess dietary proteins and sugars beyond what the body can use at the time can be turned into fat. The body even has the ability to convert excess hormones like insulin into extra fat. The original plan was that this stored fuel would be used during lean times to keep us functioning.

It took thousands of years to develop this system, and it isn't going to change any time soon. In the meantime, it took a much shorter period for us to come up with some much more efficient ways of providing ourselves with food, effectively eliminating the feast/famine cycle in many parts of the world. Not surprisingly, these are the same parts of the world that are now struggling with obesity problems.

2

Hormones, Proteins and
Fat Burning

Tammy is an incredible lady. She has a full-time career as a radio producer, and a part-time career as a professional announcer and radio host. She is fun loving and dedicated to her daily workout. In fact, Tammy never misses her evening Boxersize classes for fear of gaining extra weight. She's tried almost every diet ever invented, and even thought up a couple of her own. All failed miserably.

About one year ago, Tammy came to see me about her frustrations over never-ending diets and her continual increase in weight. After carefully reviewing the foods she ate, her exercise routine and taking a fat-percentage measurement, I recognized that Tammy was eating too many processed carbohydrates and not getting enough dietary proteins. Tammy was also doing the wrong kind of exercise. All this made it likely that the main reason why Tammy couldn't lose her extra fat was because she had a high resting insulin level, a problem in common with millions of over-fat people around the world.

I suggested that she reduce her consumption of processed carbohydrates, replace them with more dietary proteins and carbohydrates that were not highly processed (such as whole grains, vegetables and fruit), and even add in some essential fats, especially the omega-3s. Tammy was encouraged to eat more frequently and to add a couple of high-protein shakes as snacks between main meals. If that wasn't enough, I also suggested that Tammy cut down on her aerobic exercise and replace it with resistance training (using weights) two or three times a week.

Needless to say, none of these suggestions made any sense to Tammy. "Carbohydrates don't make me fat! How could they? They don't contain any fat to begin with!" And "You want me to eat five or six meals a day! How do you think I got fat in the first place?" To add insult to injury, "You want me to cut down on my fat-burning exercise and bulk up with weights!" Did Tammy follow my advice? Not a chance! It went counter to everything she had ever heard about losing weight.

Now fast-forward almost one year. My phone rings. "Brad, it's Tammy. Guess what?" The pitch of her voice was rising in excitement. "I've lost nearly 20 pounds and it's all due to your advice!" Tammy proceeded to tell me that she had literally come to her wits' end almost two months earlier. "If I'd gained just one more pound on another crummy diet and exercise plan, I would have killed myself," she said.

In desperation, Tammy remembered my advice from months earlier. Figuring she had failed at every other weight-loss approach, she decided to give it a go. In just a few days, after lowering her refined carbs and switching to weight training, Tammy could hardly believe it as the fat started melting off. Twenty pounds of energy-sapping fat are gone, and it's still coming off as this book goes to print.

Tammy is not the exception; she's the rule! Millions of frustrated and confused men and women with the same outdated beliefs regarding weight loss are in search of the truth. Unfortunately, they cling to the old views that research and years of continual weight-loss failure have shown will not work, and never will.

OUR GENES, OUR FATHER'S GENES, OUR GREAT-GREAT-GREAT-GREAT ...

We've all heard the saying "you are what you eat." Well, when it comes to how our fat cells behave, we also are what our ancestors ate. According to Dr. Boyd Eaton, an expert in evolution and the diet of early humans, 99% of our genetic structure was formed before our biological ancestors evolved into Homo sapiens (about 40,000 years ago), and 99.99% of our genes were formed before the advent of agriculture (about 10,000 years ago).

Our genes have evolved through millions of years that have shaped our need for specific nutrients. In fact, our genes—which control every function in our bodies—are essentially the same as those of our early ancestors. If we feed these genes well, they will do their job well, which ultimately means keeping us healthy. But if we give these genes nutrients that they are unfamiliar with, nutrients that were not part of their history or nutrients that are in the wrong ratios, our genes will eventually malfunction, which leads to disease.

So, just what did our ancestors eat? A diet far different from what we are eating today. We are consumers of a modern diet rich in refined carbohydrates and overprocessed dietary fats. Genetically, we are prepared for a diet of wild game and unprocessed fruits and vegetables. Things *have* changed in the last 100 centuries. In this time we have lost touch with the fundamental principles that shaped our physiology and gone beyond the capabilities of the genes that got us this far in the first place. Instead of eating like our ancestors, we have become carbohydrate addicts. We are consuming carbohydrates as our main source of food, with dietary proteins as the supplement. Dr. Eaton also has stated, through extensive research, that the early human diet consisted of at least 30% protein. So what does this have to do with obesity? A lot!

According to geneticists, it takes almost 100,000 years for any substantial genetic alterations to become part of our cells. Since we've been consuming carbohydrates as our main food source for only 10,000 years, it may take another 90,000 years for our genes to catch up with a high-carbohydrate diet. Dr. Eaton believes that the less we eat like our ancestors, the more susceptible we'll be to many of the diseases of modern civilization, diseases such as diabetes, heart disease, arthritis and cancer.

In order to get beyond the Fat Wars and work with our bodies for health, we must eat what our bodies are genetically receptive to. Since our hunter-gatherer brothers and sisters from centuries ago functioned best on a diet rich in proteins from lean meat, supplemented with whole fruits and vegetables, we would be wise to do the same. Just as Charles Darwin taught us, the forces of natural selection allowed us to evolve to function optimally on these foods. And since food was not always in abundance, and we didn't have the convenience or guarantee of at least three balanced meals per day, we developed an incredible storage capacity within our 30 billion fat cells. Don't forget: each and every one of those 30 billion fat cells can expand 1,000 times in volume, and if that isn't enough, they can also increase in number.

HORMONE ONE: INSULIN, A DOUBLE AGENT

The body has many hormones at work—nearly 30 that we know of (with many more to be found)—but only a few are involved in fat gain and loss. Insulin, a chemical protein-based hormone that is secreted from the pancreas immediately following a meal and during periods of elevated blood sugar, is a key one. Insulin is the Dr. Jekyll and Mr. Hyde of metabolism. On the positive side, insulin performs functions necessary for life, including the deposit of sugar (glycogen) in muscle so we have an ample source of energy, and the synthesis of chemical proteins for building enzymes, hormones and muscle. But the negative side of insulin is that when it's produced in excess, it plays a major role in obesity, as well as cardiovascular disease and Type 2 diabetes.

Insulin and Diabetes

When most of us think of insulin, we tend to think of diabetes. There are actually many types of diabetes. Type 1, which has been referred to as juvenile diabetes, accounts for only 10% of the disorder known as diabetes. Type 1 diabetes is due to a dysfunction of the pancreas, which is unable to secrete either any or enough insulin.

Type 2 diabetes is a whole different problem, accounting for almost 90% of people with diabetes. Type 2 diabetes, or adult-onset diabetes, is caused when the insulin receptor sites on the cells become insensitive to the hormone. When insulin cannot bind to the cell to allow the sugar to enter it, blood sugar can't leave the bloodstream. Instead, both blood sugar and blood insulin levels remain elevated. (Impaired glucose tolerance is a precondition of diabetes and affects many more people than those with diabetes. Again, the blood cells that store the blood sugar as glycogen don't work well with insulin. The transport proteins inside the cells that help bring in the sugar are working at a slow pace, and more insulin is needed to push the sugar into the cells.)

Insulin and Fat Storage

Because insulin is especially sensitive to dietary carbohydrates—they are metabolized into sugar—the more carbohydrates we eat at one time, especially the refined kinds, the greater the amount of insulin is needed to clear sugar from the bloodstream. And here's the kicker—insulin is the major factor in fat-storage.

In terms of fat burning (and storage) high insulin levels biochemically reduce the levels of a hormone-sensitive, fat-release enzyme called Lipoprotein Lipase. Conversely, low insulin levels increase levels of a hormone called glucagon, which mobilizes fat so the enzyme carriers can transport it into the muscle cells for fuel. In other words, when insulin levels are high, the body can't access fat for energy—excess insulin makes us fat and keeps us fat! In order to free up the fat so it can be burned in the muscle cells, we've got to lower our insulin levels.

So just how do we lower our insulin levels? By changing our diet and exercising properly. We can also try supplementing our diet by taking certain nutrients that increase insulin sensitivity (see Chromium in Chapter 12).

Many scientists, physicians and weight loss experts believe the key to successful long-term fat loss is in balancing our insulin levels, lowering our glucose load and increasing our protein intake. You may be thinking, "Well, I don't eat much sugar and I'm still fat." Here's a little statistic to put things into a better perspective: According to the best-selling book *Sugar Busters*, "Most North Americans consume approximately one cup of sugar daily, that's almost 150 pounds of sugar each year." Also, virtually every carbohydrate we consume (bagels, potatoes, carrots and breads) is quickly metabolized into glucose (sugar) in our systems. The higher our glucose load, the higher our insulin levels. Understanding how insulin levels relate to increased fat gain will give us the knowledge to keep our 30 billion fat cells from growing exponentially.

HORMONE TWO: HUMAN GROWTH HORMONE

One of growth hormone's main jobs is to regulate growth, especially at puberty, but its role goes much beyond that. Human growth hormone (HGH) is also responsible for increasing lean body mass (muscle), and decreasing stored body fat by freeing it up as an energy source.

HGH is secreted in rhythmic pulses from the pituitary gland in the centre of our brain throughout the day and night, but primarily while we sleep. In fact, up to 75% of HGH is produced while we are in our deepest phase of sleep (stages III and IV). It is also produced in response to intense exercise (especially resistance training). The pulsing effect of HGH is regulated by two opposing hormones produced in the hypothalamus, a gland that sits just above the pituitary. One of these hormones is responsible for increasing the amount of HGH in the bloodstream; the second hormone is responsible for decreasing or halting the production of HGH.

The pattern of HGH secretion is roughly as follows:
- 7 a.m. – low
- 9 a.m. – medium
- 11 a.m. – low
- Noon – high
- 2–5 p.m. – low and medium peaks
- 7 p.m. – medium/high
- Midnight – large bursts (if asleep by 9 p.m.)
- 3–6 a.m. – small peaks

Three factors emerge in achieving optimal natural secretions: to bed early with sound sleep from 11 p.m.–2 a.m.; doing regular strenuous exercise; and remaining free of disease.

HGH only hangs around for a few minutes after it's pumped into our bloodstream. Although its appearance is fleeting, it is very powerful. In those few minutes, growth hormone has a mission—it must make its way to two locations. One is the fat cells, where it latches onto specific growth hormone receptors, activating the release of stored fat for energy. The other location is the liver, where it stimulates the release of a special set of hormones called insulin-like growth factors (IGF) or somatomedins. (These growth factors bear a close resemblance in structure to insulin, thus their names. The various somatomedins are required for the growth of the cells, bones, muscles, organs and the immune system. Even though HGH stimulates the release of these growth factors, they are also created independently.)

HGH on the Decline

After our early twenties, HGH declines approximately 14% per decade; around the age of 60 we have experienced an 80% decline in the hormone. IGF levels follow closely behind with a decline of nearly 50% soon after middle age (40). It is widely believed that these prodigious declines of HGH and IGF are directly responsible for not only robbing us of our youth, but for the body transformation that we have all come to fear.

By retirement age, nearly two-thirds of our population will have lost at least one-third of their muscle mass and replaced it with (you guessed it) fat. This loss of lean body mass is a biological trait shared by the majority of the population as we age.

Nature's Way to Higher HGH Levels

Nearly 50% of the pituitary gland, where HGH is produced, is comprised of growth hormone-producing cells. The amazing thing is that these cells can be stimulated to produce youthful amounts of this hormone at any age. Dr. William Sonntag and colleagues, of the Bowman Gray School of Medicine in North Carolina, recently completed a study showing that the age-related decline in HGH secretion is actually reversible. The best approach for increasing growth hormone and its growth factor family is to supply the body with ways that can increase its supply naturally. That way the body won't build up a defense mechanism that can eventually cut off the supply of this essential hormone.

Bioavailable IGF and its growth factor friends taken orally are naturally occurring and in exceptionally high concentrations in life's first food, colostrum—that first secretion of mother's milk after birth. Antiaging clinics around the world have isolated growth hormone and its growth factor family, charging exorbitant fees for something found naturally and in perfect balance in colostrum. The added benefit of colostrum is that these muscle-building, fat-burning growth factors are not degraded by our systems. Instead, they enter our bloodstreams intact. Even better news is that bovine colostrum can be found on your local health-food store shelves. Given the fact that two-thirds of our population will lose one third of their muscle by the time they are 60, we can use all the natural help we can get!

Human Growth Hormone

Many studies have demonstrated both physical and mental improvements, particularly in the elderly, following the use of HGH injections. It must be remembered, however, that there can also be side effects such as diabetes, hypoglycemia, disturbance of homeostasis and disfigurement following improper use of the hormone. Many users do not achieve the desired effects. One of the reasons is because the body will slow or even stop its natural release of the hormone by increasing its levels of the anti-growth hormone somatostatin.

Evidence of this shutdown sequence was published in an article in 1988 in the *Journal of Applied Physiology*, which followed two groups of highly trained weight lifters who had no deficiencies of growth hormone to begin with. One group was given injections of the hormone, while the other group was given placebo (containing no active substance) injections. Both groups continued weight lifting throughout the study. At the end of the study, the group that had received the hormone injection showed a significant decrease in body fat with an increase in fat-free mass (muscle), while the placebo group showed no change. However, the study also revealed that the men receiving the hormone injections had a suppression of their natural growth hormone response. HGH is not something to experiment with without the aid of an experienced physician.

HGH and Fat Burning

As you will see in Part II, the human body relies on three basic sources of energy: carbohydrates, dietary fats and dietary proteins. The carbohydrates must first be converted into glucose before the body can use them as an energy source. Excess glucose is converted into glycogen and stored, although the body can only store four or five hours' worth of glucose energy in the form of glycogen. Once a good supply of the glycogen has been used up, the body begins burning fat. At this point, the body enters a semifasting mode, and HGH is responsible for switching it into this mode.

HOW FAT IS TRANSPORTED

Blood is a "liquid organ." It is comprised of approximately 50% red blood cells and 50% liquid. The liquid is called plasma and when the clotting factor (fibrinogen) is removed, what remains is called serum, a yellowish liquid that contains hundreds of different specialized chemical proteins. The average person has approximately 3 L of serum. The serum carries the essential, life-giving substances through the blood vessels to nourish all the cells in the body. The serum also carries the waste by-products away from those cells so they don't become toxic.

One law of chemistry is really quite simple: fats and water don't mix. Blood and body fluids are almost all water. Thus, nature is presented with a problem: How to transport the lipids (fats, which include cholesterol) from one place to another? This is accomplished by a group of transport proteins called lipoproteins. Some are referred to as chylomicrons, some as low-density lipoproteins (LDLs) and others as high-density lipoproteins (HDLs). The density refers to the chemical protein content. The higher the density of the chemical protein, the healthier it is for us.

Albumin, the dominant transport protein in blood serum, is a very high-density lipoprotein (VHDL). In the simplest terms, the more of these fat-carrying transport proteins we have, particularly HDL and albumin, the better the blood is able to transport all the lipids, including cholesterol. Without these transporters, the fats would simply stick to the walls of the blood vessels and create havoc. Albumin has been called the life factor by many top researchers because the more we have, the healthier we will be and the longer we will live.

UNDERSTANDING ALBUMIN

Albumin is the most studied of all the chemical proteins. It has more than 60 roles, including the transport of nutrients and removal of wastes, maintenance of cell stability and control of DNA replication. It is also the major transporter of fatty acids. It has a special cargo-hold for three fatty acids per albumin molecule, although it normally carries only two. Under stress, it may carry up to six. The combination of albumin bound to correct types and levels of fatty acids is vital for cell growth. In the body, countless trillions of albumin molecules are continuously transporting fatty acids to and from cells and to and from the liver.

It is difficult to be fat, misshapen and unhealthy when one has optimal levels of albumin. The average person has only 40 g of albumin per liter of blood with an albumin/globulin (A/G) ratio of only 1.5. Healthy people have albumin levels of at least 50 g per liter with an A/G ratio of a minimum of 2.0. Super levels are above 55 g per liter with A/G ratio of 3.0.

Albumin Levels

The level of albumin is determined by the level of immune/inflammatory proteins. The greater the stress on the immune system, the lower the level of albumin. Every single hospital in the world has attempted to raise albumin levels with high-protein diets, supplements, even by intravenous injection. In every case, this approach fails. Only by reducing the stress on the immune system, resulting in a natural decline in antibodies and inflammatory chemical proteins, can one make more room in the blood for albumin. The liver makes trillions of albumin molecules daily. When defense proteins rise, the liver reduces production of albumin. When these proteins decline, the liver increases the production of albumin.

A New Approach to Personal Hygiene

It has become increasingly evident over the years that infections are the major cause of diseases linked to overeating or being overweight or in poor physical condition. Lower socioeconomic groups, particularly those who are elderly, are more susceptible to these problems, perhaps because of poor hygiene.

Dr. Kenneth Seaton, an Australian research scientist specializing in aging and immune function, developed the High-Performance Hygiene System to elevate albumin levels. He spent the last 20 years developing a new system of personal hygiene based on cleaning the thumb/fingernails, nasal passageway and eyes. This approach greatly reduces respiratory infections, allergies and skin problems in order to achieve optimal albumin levels, which in turn lead to improved physical health and a trim shape. Perhaps now you will understand hygiene's subtle influence over physical condition and shape.

While diet is of great importance for overall health, it is not *the* determining factor in the concentration of albumin. According to Australian researcher Dr. Kenneth Seaton, hygiene is the single-most important factor because it determines the concentration of defense/inflammatory proteins. In simple terms, the stress on the immune system is a reflection of one's standard of personal hygiene and general health (such as whether or not one smokes or has chronic disease).

Swimmers probably have the best all-round physiques (and just in case you're wondering, I'm not a swimmer). Fit, muscular people are in good shape, inside and out. This also explains why swimmers have such high levels of albumin. Exposure to sunlight and regular swimming as exercise are excellent natural hygiene habits, reducing the stress on the immune system, allowing more room in the blood for albumin.

As we know, dietary fats and cholesterol are essential for life and good health and, because they are not soluble in serum, they require transport proteins such as albumin to get to the cells. The more of these transport proteins we have, the more we are able to handle dietary fats and cholesterol. Those who maintain high levels of albumin and other carrier proteins can eat lots of dietary fats and not suffer consequences such as deposits in the blood vessels. Further, when necessary, they can generate lots of energy by efficiently utilizing the adipose tissue, quickly converting its fatty acids and transporting them to the trillions of cells throughout the body.

Human Growth Hormone and Albumin
Increasing growth hormone levels will increase the overall anabolic (muscle-building/fat-burning) activity in the body. The anabolic benefit of HGH is to increase dietary protein synthesis (the building of proteins). Proteins are assembled from hundreds of amino acids that must be present in the right amounts so they can be assembled in the right order. From approximately 20 amino acids, the body forms over 50,000 protein structures that produce muscle tissue, including skeletal, smooth and cardiac tissue; collagen; skin; hair; nails; eyes; connective tissue; cartilage; bone; neurotransmitters; hormones and enzymes.

Free amino acids in the blood serum are usually found in low concentrations (0.37 g per liter of blood). As a backup source, nature has devised a remarkable means of supplying the perfect amount of amino acids needed for assembly. This source is the protein albumin. The liver makes trillions of molecules of albumin each day.

Nutritionally human albumin is a perfect transport protein. It contains just the right balance of amino acids (needed for proper growth) for both children and adults. (Animals develop almost exclusively within the egg by using the massive amount of albumin in the white.) Without sufficient amounts of albumin, over and above that needed for transportation and other roles, protein synthesis will fail, anabolic metabolism will switch to catabolic (breakdown), and we will not be able to lose an ounce of fat.

THE BIOCHEMISTRY OF FAT BURNING

The single most important factor in achieving optimal health, fat loss and maximum life span is a slight reduction in dietary intake and an increase in energy production. I realize that this is not news. Although you already know this, pay close attention to the following paragraph. It could rocket you on to fat-loss success.

It is important to realize that the fasting period between evening and morning, if it's adequate, is probably the most effective natural way to cause beneficial secretions of HGH and its helpers, as well as free the cargo-holds on albumin. One of the reasons is because nature has scheduled the optimal production of both HGH and albumin during the nighttime sleep/ fasting mode.

Optimal fat-burning/fasting periods usually occur from the evening meal (no later than 7:30 p.m.) to breakfast at around 7 a.m., approximately 11½ hours later. Normally, during this sleep/fast period, the body switches to fat burning by around 1 a.m., provided a person goes to sleep between 9 and 10 p.m. and insulin levels are not elevated by any snacks along the way. This fasting/fat-burning cycle is excellent for health, growth, repair and slowing the aging process. Best results are obtained when this fasting period lasts for at least 14 hours, with the greatest effects of HGH being produced in 16 hours. If we drink even fruit juice, coffee or tea, we can switch the body out of the HGH-producing fasting mode back to using sugars as the main energy source. Insulin will be produced, fat burning will stop and protein synthesis will be interrupted. This is usually what's going on while we sleep.

The secret is simple yet sometimes difficult because of willpower. As stated, the evening meal should be no later than 7:30 p.m., then drink only water until the first meal the next day. Even if the fast lasts only for the normal 11½ hours each day, it is beneficial and can profoundly reduce weight and improve health. And if you follow my advice in the exercise chapters in Part III and train first thing in the morning on an empty stomach, you can increase growth hormone production and even further increase fat burning all day long.

3

His Fat

Russell turned 50 almost a month ago, and he wasn't too happy about it! Then again, why should he be happy? Russell is not the man he was 20 years ago. Gone are the days when he could stay up all night and party with his buddies. Russell now feels it the next day, even if he misses a couple of hours of sleep. And gone are the days when he would proudly tear off his shirt on a warm summer day to expose a finely tuned physique. Those muscles have been covered with layer upon layer of fat. Russell wouldn't be caught dead taking off his shirt at the beach these days. Also gone are the days when Russell actually had enough energy to go to the gym after work. Now he feels drained when he gets home, mustering only enough energy to plop himself down on the couch. Exercise is reduced to pointing and clicking his new, high-tech remote. What about sex? What about it?!

Russell's temperament has also changed. This once patient and humorous guy now snaps at almost everything. Arguments have become the norm around the house—Russell's wife and children avoid him more and more. Russell has become what every man, woman and child fears … a Fat, Grumpy, Old Man.

Russell is not alone—he's experiencing an all-too-common transition that is referred to as andropause. If the word sounds familiar, it's probably because it resembles that passage in a woman's life called menopause. (Andropause is actually called male menopause in some circles.) The word "andropause" first appeared in the literature in 1952 and is defined as the natural cessation of the sexual function in older men due to a marked reduction in male hormone levels.

Now, what do andropause and male hormones have to do with fat loss? Actually, they're the link between obesity and middle-aged men. Andropause works ever so slowly on unsuspecting guys until they wake up one morning as completely different people. The men we once knew are slowly replaced—by bigger, grumpier, flabbier ones.

IT'S MORE THAN JUST A SEX HORMONE!

Just as menopause reflects a decline in a woman's hormonal cascade, andropause reflects a decline of male hormones. Collectively, the male hormones are called androgens. At the top of the androgen list is the one we've all heard of before: testosterone. Ninety-five percent of testosterone is made in the testes, and 5% in the adrenal glands. Testosterone is a fat-soluble hormone that is synthesized from cholesterol. It's the hormone that assures the development and integrity of the genitals in males, but it also regulates the structure of all body proteins—and a whole lot more.

You thought testosterone was just a sex hormone? Wrong! Testosterone travels to every part of the human body. When naturally abundant, testosterone is at the core of energy, stamina, sexuality and a lean body. There are receptors for it from the brain to the toes. Testosterone is involved in the making of proteins, which in turn builds muscle. It's also a key player in the manufacture of bone. Testosterone improves oxygen uptake throughout the body, revitalizing all tissues, and oxygen is a fundamental ingredient in the formula for burning body fat. Testosterone also helps control blood sugar. We know it's that excess blood sugar that causes us to store fat at unprecedented rates as the insulin that controls the excess blood sugar shuts down the body's ability to access fat as a fuel source.

After about age 35, a man's testosterone levels begin to decline. This slight dip in normal levels goes unnoticed at first and causes only modest changes in body composition—maybe a slight increase in those love handles from year to year. The decline in testosterone is felt not just in the tummy area. There is also a weakening of muscle strength and bone matter. Declining testosterone secretion also causes the organs to begin to lose their function over time, resulting in changes such as memory loss and increased irritability. A man will also notice more and more fatigue-related deficiencies. But it is the noticeable increase in body fat that will sound the first alarm that things are not as they used to be.

Restoring testosterone to optimal levels has been proven to increase muscle mass (which sets the stage for a decrease in body fat); boost brain function, including memory, visual acuity and concentration; protect the heart—it reduces virtually every cardiovascular risk factor, including high cholesterol, high blood sugar, abnormal clotting and stress response; strengthens the bones and, of course, lowers insulin levels.

Testosterone and Obesity

The importance of testosterone can't be underestimated, especially in men who need to lose excess fat. An adult man's testicles normally produce 7–10 mg of testosterone per day, and testosterone is an essential hormone for fat burning. In over-fat or obese males, androgen levels decline in proportion to the degree of obesity—the lower the level of testosterone, the fatter the man becomes, and visa versa.

A newly discovered hormone called leptin, which is produced by the body's fat cells, is believed to be a major culprit here. Leptin circulates in the bloodstream at concentrations equal to the amount of fat reserves—the higher the body's fat content, the higher the levels of leptin. Leptin can actually inhibit testosterone production. (This may be one of the reasons why over-fat and obese boys often experience a delay in reaching puberty.)

The decline in testosterone goes hand in hand with the decline in muscle mass, which ultimately results in a slowdown in men's anabolic (tissue-building) metabolism. In the never-ending battle to control the slowdown of metabolism, adequate levels of testosterone are critical for slowing down the deterioration of fat-burning engines. We all know the importance of muscle when it comes to fat burning—the gradual loss of testosterone that comes with aging compounds the problem of excess fat by decreasing the amount of fat-burning muscle even more.

Swedish researchers R. Rosmond and P. Björntorp, in a 1998 study of 284 middle-aged men, discovered that low testosterone levels were indirectly or directly related to the amount of fat the men were carrying around their midsections. Those with too much fat around their abdomens were more likely to have major health problems like diabetes and heart disease. The Lipid Research Center in Ste-Foy, Quebec, did a 1997 study involving 76 men, showing that the higher the testosterone levels, the better the levels of good cholesterol (HDL) and the lower the levels of bad cholesterol (LDL). This same study showed that men with higher testosterone levels also had lower levels of triglycerides (the fats that travel around our bloodstream and are all too easily stored as body fat). Rosmond and Björntorp's 1998 study of 51-year-old men found that obese men were more likely to be anxious and depressed.

Testosterone and Exercise

In 1996, the *New England Journal of Medicine* reported on a study involving three groups of men. One group was given testosterone and prescribed a strength-training program, the second group was given testosterone and told not to exercise, and the third group did the strength-training program without testosterone. To no one's surprise, the group that exercised on testosterone gained the most muscle and lost the most fat, *but* the group that took testosterone without exercise had greater improvement in muscle and fat composition than the group that trained without it.

There is a lot of research on the effects of proper exercise when it comes to raising testosterone naturally. The misconception is that aerobic exercise is the best exercise of all. The truth of the matter is that the only exercise that has been shown in studies to raise testosterone levels effectively is weight-resistant exercise.

Testosterone in Chains

We certainly can't ignore the research when it comes to the fat-fighting potential of testosterone, but not all testosterone is created equal. Not all the testosterone in the body is biologically active. It is only the free, unbound testosterone that exerts its wondrous effects on men's bodies. It is also the free, physiologically active testosterone that declines the most with age. In a 1999 Belgian study involving 372 males aged 20 to 85, decreased levels of free testosterone went along with increased body mass index ratings and increased fat mass. The younger the subjects, the lower the fat levels and the higher the amounts of muscle tissue. This study also indicated that the younger subjects had much higher free testosterone levels than the older ones, and researchers concluded that free testosterone positively influenced body composition.

Free testosterone declines with age because of a specific protein, called sex hormone-binding globulin or SHBG, which binds with it. Testosterone is unable to do its powerful fat-burning work once it is bound. It is not uncommon for free testosterone to decline by about 1% per year after the age of 40. In a 1998 Greek study involving 52 elderly men, it was discovered that the increase in SHBG was directly related to the increase in the chronological age of the men. On average, there was a 13% increase in the chemical protein per five years, making it harder and harder for elderly men to lose weight.

PUMP UP THE VOLUME!

The solution seems obvious: men need to bring their testosterone levels back to what they were when they were lean and firm and happy.

Set It Free Naturally

Well, nature works in mysterious ways and can offer us a powerful alternative to artificial substances, which often have a number of side effects. We are not talking about using testosterone injections to burn body fat. Instead, we are talking about using what is already in our bodies in the first place.

One natural herb offers us this potential without side effects—*Urtica dioica*, but you may have heard of it before under its more common name, stinging nettle. In a paper published in 1995 in *Planta Medica*, a proprietary extract of the stinging nettle plant was shown to prevent the SHBG from latching onto the cell membrane of the prostate gland. According to this and other studies, stinging nettle extract is not only a powerful testosterone helper, it can also help to prevent and perhaps even treat prostate disease.

When it comes to increasing the fat-burning effects of testosterone, a particular extract of the stinging nettle plant is showing great promise. Special compounds in stinging nettle extract (known as lignans) have a very high affinity to SHBG. Researchers have been studying the beneficial effects of plant lignans on hormone-dependent cancers for some time now. These lignans are able to bind to SHBG in place of testosterone. In effect, the bound testosterone gets thrown off the SHBG—freed to exert its physiological effects on the body.

There are many different forms of stinging nettle available on the market, but it is only the newer extracts that are proving to be extremely powerful testosterone helpers. Many of the stinging nettle products on the market today have been extracted using alcohol or ethanol. These extraction processes either don't do the optimum job, or, in some cases, they don't do the job at all. As you will note throughout *Fat Wars*, newer and better processes have been developed for most extracts; look for products that have either aqueous (water) or methanolic extracts. In this case, the difference could literally make or break the testosterone connection.

Artificial Testosterone vs Natural Testosterone

In Europe, a number of safe and effective methods of testosterone replacement have existed for years. Until the recent release of the testosterone patch and the newer topical delivery creams, the choices in the United States and Canada have been limited. Prescription options have included either injection or the oral route.

Even though natural testosterone has been available since 1938, it has not been widely prescribed. Most of the anabolic (tissue-building) steroids that are responsible for the negative publicity surrounding testosterone are actually synthetic analogs of natural testosterone. When taken orally in large quantities, they are potentially dangerous and can cause serious liver diseases, as well as organ failure.

When testosterone is taken orally, it is rapidly metabolized by the liver, so injectable preparations of esters, which are more fat soluble, were produced to ensure a longer life span in the body. Testosterone esters, which are more lipid soluble, are injected in a peanut-oil base to increase the half-life of the testosterone. One injection can maintain normal serum levels of testosterone for 10–14 days. Some of these esters include: testosterone propionate, testosterone cypionate and testosterone enanthate.

Testosterone can also be delivered via testosterone patches and creams. Natural testosterone, synthesized in a laboratory into an exact molecular duplicate to our own natural endogenous testosterone, can be taken safely in larger doses by men who have a testosterone deficiency. These higher doses of natural testosterone seem to present no apparent health risks. Some of these new pharmaceutical prescriptions are:

- Testoderm®, a patch-delivery system of natural testosterone
- Androderm®, a similar preparation that can be applied anywhere
- A new dihydroxytestosterone gel is presently being developed, as well as newer creams that can deliver natural testosterone very effectively.

It is important to mimic the natural secretion pattern of testosterone in the human body when applying any patches, creams or gels. Testosterone levels naturally peak early in the morning, so application should follow this routine. It is also important to work closely with a medical professional for both evaluation and treatment with any form of testosterone, natural or synthetic, as it's a very powerful substance.

NATURAL TESTOSTERONE DISCOVERY

Elk velvet antler or EVA, an extract from an elk antler, is finally becoming known in the West. Extracts of EVA have been used in Asia for over 2000 years to treat a myriad of disorders. The extract is a living biological factory loaded with some of the most incredible substances in their natural synergistic ratios, including amino acids, essential for anabolic metabolism; growth hormones, plus a whole array of growth factors and their precursors; and natural anti-inflammatory agents known as prostaglandins (most disease is associated with an increase in inflammatory messengers). Research reports on the benefits of EVA, coming from all over the world, are numerous, but one of the most exciting studies was performed in 1998 at the University of Alberta. This study showed that a specific extract of EVA, taken orally, can significantly boost the testosterone levels in the body.

MEN ARE FROM ... VENUS?!

Losing testosterone or having it bound up as a man ages are far from the only problems he faces. As men experience a drop in their testosterone levels, or a rise in their SHBG levels, they usually experience a rise in their estrogen levels too. In men as well as postmenopausal women, most estrogens are produced directly from androgens (male hormones). Androgens and estrogens have similar metabolic effects in the liver where enzymes convert testosterone into estradiol or E2, a form of estrogen.

> There are actually three subtypes of estrogen in the body: estrone (E1), estradiol (E2—the active "female hormone") and estriol (E3). Estriol is the protective estrogen of the body, and its deficiency directly causes the hot flashes and nervousness associated with menopause in women.
>
> Estradiol is responsible for a great deal of the mayhem inflicted on the aging male body. The conversion of androgens to estrogens is called aromatization and is carried out by the enzyme aromatase. Aromatase is a very powerful partner in fat storing because most of this enzyme resides in, of all places, the fat cells. The more fat cells, and the larger those fat cells become, the more aromatase they manufacture, and the less testosterone men have for fat loss.

As men age, they lose muscle and gain fat. The more fat, the higher the conversion of testosterone to estrogen. The less testosterone men have, the less muscle they make. In order to effectively increase the amount of natural testosterone in the body, men must also look at inhibiting this conversion of testosterone into estrogen. Once again nature provides us with a number of powerful ways to help prevent this conversion from taking place.

- In addition to inhibiting SHBG binding, stinging nettle root has also been shown to inhibit testosterone-conversion activity.
- Soy isoflavones have been shown to inhibit conversion activity.
- One of the most powerful conversion inhibitors to date is a bioflavonoid called chrysin. Chrysin was shown to be similar in both potency and effectiveness to the conversion-inhibiting drug, aminoglutethimide.

It is not uncommon for a man of retirement age to have higher estrogen levels in his body than a woman of the same age, provided that the woman isn't on estrogen therapy, so it stands to reason that the natural compounds available today to boost free testosterone may soon be a staple of any man's war on fat gain.

4

Her Fat

A woman's body is designed to store fat. More than a man's?! *Yes.*
Recent research has demonstrated that women's fat cells are different from
men's in both look and performance. As a matter of fact, when researchers
analyzed women's and men's fat cells, this is what they discovered:
- women's fat cells are up to five times larger than men's
- women's fat cells can contain up to twice the fat-storing
  enzymes
- women's fat cells can contain half the fat-releasing enzymes

What does this mean? It means it's easier for women to put on fat,
and it's harder for women to take it off. This is not fair. In terms of evolution and survival, it is, however, what worked. Evolution's priorities
are not the same as ours. Women will have to work with what they've been
given here.

The odds in the Fat Wars are stacked against women from the start.
We know that muscle is the metabolic engine of the body that causes us to
burn fat, and men carry, on average, forty pounds more muscle than women
do. Men also produce ten times more testosterone than women do—testosterone is a muscle-building, fat-burning hormone. Men manufacture up to
twice the amount of fat-releasing enzymes than women do. The more of
these enzymes, the faster fat is released as fuel.

All of these factors give men a higher metabolism than women have.
They can burn, on average, 30% more calories during exercise than women
can. To add insult to injury, they can burn on average up to 30% more
calories while at rest.

AND THEN THERE'S ESTROGEN

Testosterone is a fat-burning hormone; estrogen is not. Estrogen is a group of three hormones that regulate women's reproductive functions. (See page 30 in Chapter 3 for a full description.) Estrogen is also known to perform over 300 different functions in the body, which affect everything from building bones to strengthening the heart. It is now suggested that estrogen also works on regulating the brain.

Estrogen is normally produced by a woman's ovaries and, to a lesser extent, by the adrenal glands. As women age, estrogen production from the ovaries and glands starts to dwindle. Hormones are the messengers of the body, and the body considers losing any of them as a big deal. Over time, women's genetics have built in some clever ways to deal with this decrease. As the hormone levels drop, the body is making plans for future estrogen manufacturing sites, and the best location seems to be Fat Central.

A woman's body senses the need to start shifting estrogen production sometime in her mid-thirties. Now known as perimenopause, this is a period of very long, gradual transition that can actually last for up to 20 years—from the mid- to late thirties for the majority of women, ending in their mid-fifties. It is the ever-so-slight hormone changes that affect a woman's cycle, including her mood swings and her weight. As Debra Waterhouse puts it in her book, *Outsmarting the Female Fat Cell*, "it is during these transitional years that a woman's body goes from that of an hourglass shape to a beer glass." Whoa!

Once estrogen levels decline to a certain point, fat-storing enzymes are increased and fat-releasing enzyme activity is slowed down or stopped all together. The fat cells are getting ready to store, store and store some more, getting ready to become estrogen-producing factories as a woman gets older.

In case all this activity isn't enough to ensure sufficient fat cells for alternate estrogen production, women's fat cells also divide to create more. Fat cells only divide at select times in a person's lifetime, and perimenopause is one of them. Yes, fat cells begin to split, ensuring the body will have an ample supply of estrogen for the coming years.

LOCATION, LOCATION, LOCATION

In younger women, extra fat seems to find its way (no map needed here) to the buttocks, hips and thighs much too easily. But as time goes by, as a female's hormonal system declines, fat seems to become more preoccupied with one location.

The first thing a realtor is taught in real estate investing is that the better the location, the higher the returns. The female body understands the same principle—the area chosen for fat storing is the tummy area. This also happens to be the area most conducive to the production of estrogen. Fat cells located in the midsection insulate the liver and the adrenal glands, and it is with the aid of these two that estrogen is produced. The production assembly goes like this:

- the adrenal glands produce a type of testosterone (yes, the male hormone)
- the liver produces an enzyme that is necessary for the conversion of testosterone to estrogen
- the fat cells closest to the adrenal glands and the liver become the manufacturing plants for the estrogen

All in all, it's a very sophisticated estrogen-manufacturing system that has evolved over millennia to ensure women's survival into old age.

To make sure that this manufacturing process goes off without a hitch, the female body does away with unnecessary metabolic machinery. After all, there is no need to burn fat when it is needed in larger quantities for estrogen production. To secure the fat, after the age of 35 or so, the female body loses approximately one-half pound of muscle—the key metabolic engine of the body—a year. The loss of this metabolic machinery gives the female body the ability to gain at least one-and-a-half pounds of fat each year to take its place. And, no surprises here, from her mid-thirties, the typical North American woman often gains one-and-a-half pounds of extra fat each year.

Women and Testosterone

Women need healthy levels of testosterone throughout their lives. Testosterone is involved in their bodies' ability to utilize protein and manufacture bone mass. It improves oxygen uptake and helps control blood sugar. It helps regulate cholesterol and maintain a powerful immune system. Testosterone also appears to help with mental concentration and improve mood swings by maintaining a better hormonal balance.

Normal levels of testosterone are especially important for premenopausal and menopausal women. As women age, their production of testosterone also drops or becomes bound to body proteins. The loss of testosterone will show in bone loss (osteoporosis), as well as in a loss of energy, libido and muscle mass.

The larger these fat cells become, the more estrogen can be produced. This process is perfecting itself more and more each year for a woman from her mid-thirties onward. Research performed at the University of Pittsburgh showed that women who developed the largest fat cells produced at least 40% more estrogen than those with smaller ones.

I CAN'T STOP EATING!

Just because all that fat-storing capacity is in place doesn't mean that women have to take advantage of it. But wait! Another cruel trick of biology is about to kick in. Women seem to crave extra calories with increased age. Why is this? Because the declining hormone levels are wreaking havoc all round. The brain is the chief communicating organ of the body, responsible for the regulation of every body system. As the levels of estrogen drop below normal, the levels of certain chemical messengers in the brain also start to decline, including the key regulator of hunger: serotonin.

Serotonin is a neurotransmitter responsible for normal mood, behavior and feelings of satisfaction. When serotonin levels are low, we feel tired, moody and hungry. If we were hungry for vegetables it wouldn't be so bad, but the hunger cravings are for sweets. The sugars from these foods can enhance the levels of serotonin, so to keep the brain happy, women eat and eat and eat until the brain is satisfied (which doesn't last for long). In the meantime, they've added more calories that they don't physically need—so those calories go into storage. (No doubt that was the plan.)

AND NOW THE GOOD NEWS ...

There are benefits hidden in all this new fat—estrogen can now be produced to balance the negative effects of menopause.

Here's how the estrogen produced from fat cells helps women during menopause:
- it cuts the level of hot flashes to half of what leaner women experience
- it allows for better sleep
- it maintains natural collagen production so skin stays healthy
- it cuts the risk of osteoporosis to half the levels that thinner women experience

The question is: Can women find alternative estrogen without having to pack their fat cells?

ESTROGEN-MANUFACTURING PLANTS!

Menopause doesn't just happen to North American women. How do women in the rest of the world deal with it? For millennia Asian women have stayed slim into their later years without any discomfort. They consume soy.

When we refer to soy, we are referring to the components of the soybean itself, specifically phytoestrogens, which are plant compounds that contain estrogen-like molecules that have the ability to occupy the same receptor sites as our own hormones. "Phyto" means plant, and "estrogens" refer to the ability of these plant chemicals to mimic the effects of estrogen in the body. There are already over 300 plants that are known to contain these substances, with many more likely to be found in this decade.

These phytoestrogens prevent the binding of more potent estrogens, all the while emitting weak signals to the body. These signals are between 1/100, to 1/1,000 the strength of the estrogen the body produces.

Phytoestrogens have been shown to protect the body in a multitude of ways, including reducing the severity of hot flashes, irritability, mood swings and anxiety. They can also lower heart disease risk by lowering levels of the bad cholesterol (LDL), and significantly lower the risk of osteoporosis and breast cancer. As a matter of fact, Japanese women who consume these phytoestrogens in soy products have a whopping 400% lower risk of breast cancer than North American women have. Japanese women also have the highest life expectancy in the world, and are known as the healthiest women in the world. Could it be that they just have superior genes? Perhaps, if it weren't for the fact that once these women adopt our Western eating styles, they become just as susceptible as we are to these major diseases.

Our main interest is in one of the most exciting influences of phytoestrogens: their ability to help us lose fat. (Or help us not to gain it in the first place.) By eating more of these plant compounds, women can reduce the amount of fat that enters their fat cells, due to the extra estrogen the body senses.

FEELING SOY MUCH BETTER!

One of the best ways to incorporate this cellular insurance into the daily regimen is to consume more soy products, as Japanese women do. Soy products come in a multitude of forms. The most valuable are properly fermented products like firm tofu, miso or tempeh that maintain their essential phytochemicals. When it comes to the powerful effects of phytochemicals, the magic seems to lie in a class of compounds called isoflavones. Soy contains many isoflavones, but the three that are the most beneficial so far are genestein, diadzein and glycitin. It is these isoflavones that have been thoroughly researched and are responsible for soy's incredible powers.

> **Genestein**
> Genestein is actually molecularly similar in structure to the hormone estrogen, but it exhibits only 1/1,000th the activity. As a woman's estrogen hormone production declines (post-hysterectomy, menopause), genestein can elicit a beneficial weak estrogenic effect (making up for some of the deficit). But when the body is experiencing an unhealthy high level of estrogen, genestein can help blunt the effects of the excess hormone by competing for estrogen receptors that lie on the cells' (as in breast cells) surfaces.

A Note of Caution: Although there are many benefits to consuming high-quality soy and its isoflavone family, one must err on the side of caution regarding its use by pregnant women and newborns. Several animal studies in the U.S. and Finland have indicated a possible risk associated with a high intake of phytoestrogens during pregnancy, postnatal and lactation periods. These studies show a possible inhibition of the sexual development of the newborn.

Approximately one-quarter of bottle-fed children in the U.S. receive soy-based formula, which is more than is the case in other parts of the Western world. It is estimated that an infant fed exclusively on soy formula receives the estrogenic equivalent (based on body weight) of at least five birth control pills per day. By contrast, almost no phytoestrogens have been detected in dairy-based infant formula or in human milk, even when the mother consumes soy products. Until more research is completed in this area, please be cautious when considering the use of soy-based formulas and foods for your infant.

Because the phytoestrogens and isoflavones are located in the protein fraction of the soybean almost exclusively, manufacturers have been developing new technologies to isolate and create a new class of dietary protein powders, rich in phytoestrogens and isoflavones. Buyer beware! Not all of these products are created equal. The quality of the soy protein can make all the difference in its active isoflavone content. Many soy proteins are poorly produced, using an alcohol extraction method that removes most, if not all, of the active isoflavones. Many mass-produced soy products, including tofu, also lose vast amounts of their isoflavones during processing.

Traditional Japanese fermented soy foods retain their isoflavone content, and even enhance their activity. When it comes to soy protein powders, only water-extracted soy protein isolate will retain its natural isoflavone advantage. See Appendix II for recommendations on choosing an appropriate supplement.

When purchasing these new dietary protein powders, also make sure they are non-GMO certified. This means they are non-genetically modified organisms. Without going into detail about the possible future problems associated with genetically modified products, suffice it to say that they are genetically manipulated to create greater yields for the farmer. As a by-product of this manipulation, GMOs become highly unnatural organisms and as such they are less likely to have a chemical structure our bodies can deal with.

5

Baby Fat

Kids are not only growing up faster than ever, they're also growing *out* faster. Childhood obesity is reaching epidemic proportions in many developed and underdeveloped countries. Kids are taking their parents' lead and putting on the pounds of fat at an astonishing rate—and they're likely to keep them for a lifetime. Obese teens have a greater than 50% chance of becoming obese adults. If they have an obese parent, the odds climb to 80%. Statistics show that more than 30% of our children are over-fat, and one in five is considered obese.

If you have a significantly over-fat or obese child, or if you are obese and are worried that your kids will follow suit, remember that the same conditions (and the same solutions) will apply to both of you. The right foods, physical activity and recovery are also the keys to solving the problem of over-fat kids. But kids are kids, and they need your know-how (and your good example) to help them make the right choices, which means they may need a kick in the pants from time to time just to keep them on track. As a parent, your responsibility for helping your kids get on the right path lies in your ability to set a prime example.

Again, the concern is not cosmetic. The health of millions of kids is at stake. We know that being over-fat plays a huge role in the development of Type 2 diabetes. This form of diabetes used to be called adult-onset diabetes because only adults got it, but today there is an emerging epidemic of Type 2 diabetes in youngsters.

WHERE DOES IT BEGIN?

It turns out that the seeds for obesity can actually be sown in the womb. Fat cells can divide during the third trimester of pregnancy and have been shown to be very susceptible to increased insulin levels. Too much of the wrong carbohydrates during gestation can cause insulin to be secreted in response to sugars in the bloodstream. Studies have been done on mothers' blood sugar and the effect of elevated levels of glucose on gestating fetuses. Those whose mother's blood sugar had the highest readings were markedly obese by six years of age. This had nothing to do with the mother's weight during pregnancy. The offspring of diabetic mothers have been shown to exhibit unusual patterns of fat growth:

- the baby is unusually fat at birth
- the baby assumes normal weight by the first year
- fat starts to slowly accumulate on the youngster's body over the next several years
- fat accumulation begins to accelerate at year five (girls) or six (boys)
- by age eight, both male and female offspring of diabetic mothers are considered obese according to medical standards

It is believed that the mother's insulin is unable to cross the placenta and cause any problem in the developing fetus, but insulin itself may not be the problem. Insulin injected into insulin-dependent diabetic mothers has been shown to raise insulin antibodies, which do cross the placenta. Once in the fetus, these insulin antibodies are able to increase the rate at which fat cells expand and split. This and other research is showing the link between diet during early pregnancy and the effect it may have on fat metabolism later in life.

Over or Under: Which Is Worse?

Just as overeating and increasing carbohydrate consumption during pregnancy sets the stage for obesity later in life, undernourishment during pregnancy may pose its own threats. For example, in a study of mothers who experienced caloric deprivation at a critical period during pregnancy, their sons were found to experience twice the normal incidence of obesity by the age of 19. Children whose mothers smoked during pregnancy were also found to be undernourished and similar numbers of them were obese by the end of their teen years.

Researchers once believed that an excessive number of fat cells in the young were only formed during overfeeding. This theory was disproved by a series of animal studies. In one of those studies, pigs that were undernourished from ten days to one year eventually became very fat. These pigs had a normal number of fat cells at ten days of age, but these fat cells were deflated in a sense and did not register by conventional cell counting at one year. But as soon as a good amount of food was supplied, the pigs' fat cells inflated like balloons, and they became extremely fat. Not only that, but the longer the period of deprivation, the fatter they tended to become once it was over.

BOTTLES OF FAT

The baby formula industry is a big player in the Fat Wars, and it's not on the Lean Team. The further away we get from our own natural food source— that homegrown milk produced in the mother's mammary factory—the more likely it is we will flirt with obesity later in life. A 1993 study at Case Western Reserve University's School of Medicine compared rat pups that were fed a milk-substitute formula containing a majority of carbohydrates (56% of calories) with mother-fed controls who got milk containing only small amounts (8% of calories). The formula-fed rats became over-fat. It is the source of calories, not the total caloric intake during the suckling period, that can exert long-lasting effects on fat metabolism in later years, leading to the development of obesity.

Dr. K. Dewey and colleagues at the University of California found that the longer a mother breast-fed and delayed the introduction of solid food, the better the protection against adult obesity. Ninety-five percent of the obese had not been breast-fed. Breast-fed infants have been shown to be leaner than formula-fed infants at one year of age. Formula-fed infants were fatter because carbohydrates are much higher in commercial baby formulas, increasing the energy intake and causing an increase in insulin. The verdict is in—early exposure to a high-carbohydrate diet predisposes a child to over-fatness and obesity later in life.

PUBERTY PAUSE

Excess insulin and carbohydrate overindulgence in early childhood can affect our bodies later in life; one potential impact is the acceleration of the transition period between childhood and adulthood. Epidemiological research has proven that the average age of puberty in women has dropped by four to six years in the past 100 years. A century ago, the average pubescent female was 17. Now, our little girls are becoming women between the ages of 11 to 13. Early teen sexuality, not to mention the risk of early pregnancy, are obvious social results, but obesity is another.

Obesity researcher Dr. Douglas L. Foster reported in a 1995 experimental biology meeting that the levels of glucose (sugar) in our blood are the real culprits when it comes to the early onset of puberty. In his research, Dr. Foster was able to delay puberty in sheep by reducing the levels of blood glucose, and he was able to induce early puberty by increasing the levels. This precipitous reduction in the age of puberty closely approximates the major increase in the dietary consumption of high-carbohydrate diets in the last century. Many parents complain that their children, especially girls, are growing up too quickly. With the link made between a high-carbohydrate diet and early puberty, we now have another piece to the sugar puzzle.

KIDS AND FAT WARS

Early childhood is the most critical period for establishing anti-fat eating habits. What if there is one over-fat child and two of normal weight in the same family? This doesn't mean the over-fat child should be deprived while the others enjoy unlimited French fries, colas and sweet cereals. All children need to develop a lean and healthy lifestyle and the battle must be waged as a *family*. If family members continue to indulge in fat-storing foods, take part in little or no physical activity and burn the candle at both ends, all the kids will carry this behavior into adulthood. Sooner or later, it will catch up with them. Pediatric studies suggest that obstructive sleep apnea occurs in approximately 17% of obese children and adolescents. Sleep disorders in the obese may be a major cause of learning disability and school failure, although this remains to be confirmed.

Kids want things. They want the sugar-coated cereal they see on TV every Saturday morning. They want pop during recess at school. They want the munchie combo pack while watching their favorite movies. But guess what? Parents don't have to give in to their "I gotta have it now" cries. Instead of giving them what they want, give them what they need. Parents must teach them and guide them into battle to save them from a life of obesity and poor health.

Notice how we're drinking more sugar-laden soft drinks than ever these days? Kids are especially prone to drinking high-carbohydrate drinks. These "belly wash" drinks include not only pop (like colas), but also fruit juices and other so-called "natural" drinks, loaded with added corn syrup, fructose, maltodextrins, glucose polymers, dextrose and the like. Insulin is working overtime to keep kids over-fat, and the sodas, chips, fries and candy have got to go, replaced by 1% milk or water, nuts and fruits like apples and oranges. Is it easy? No. Will kids gripe and whine? Likely. But like anything worth the time we put into it, we do what we've got to do for the health of our children.

Aren't We Going to Push Them Over the Edge?

But what about eating disorders in adolescents? Won't our intervention just drive our kids to be so conscious about their weight that they'll go too far? The answer is no, so long as we approach over-fatness in children in a non-threatening way. First, we shouldn't be so concerned about weight; instead focus on fat and how it influences their health. Fat kids are not genetic freaks. Fat kids rarely have a sluggish thyroid. Instead, fat kids eat too much of the wrong foods, and they don't get enough physical activity. Concerned parents must feed themselves and their kids the foods that will awaken the fat-burning arsenals. Kids must be discouraged from doing too much sedentary activity, such as watching television, playing video games or surfing the Internet, and encouraged to do vigorous activities that will keep them on the move.

MAKING THE CHANGE: FAT LOSS FOR KIDS

Before suddenly turning a child's life upside down and charging ahead with a Fat Wars battle plan, it's important to spend some time with an over-fat child to map it out. It takes time and effort when making lifestyle changes. Fat doesn't magically appear overnight, so no one should expect it to disappear that fast either. It will take time to introduce changes into the child's life. This is especially important with older kids.

Adolescents and teenagers need to play an active role in their personal fat-loss health plan right from the start. The first thing to remember is to never place the child on a diet of reduced calories. A child's metabolism is especially sensitive to deprivation. When their cells realize that nourishment is being cut off, the fat-storing enzymes will go into high gear. Then, when the child comes off the diet, their fat-burning enzymes, transport proteins and hormones will be so depleted that they'll easily put the fat back on, and then some. Sound familiar? Your (and your child's) mantra should be "Never diet, never diet, never diet."

LET'S GET PHYSICAL

Today's kids are less physically active than earlier generations. Most kids today catch a ride to and from school. In much of North America, gym class is a thing of the past. Many kids are brought up in a household with two working parents. In inner cities it can be risky to play outside, with an increase in crime, gangs and traffic. For these reasons, many kids go straight home from school, lock the door and turn on the TV. The hockey stick has been replaced with a video game joystick. The baseball glove has been replaced by a bag of chips. Surfing the net requires little physical exertion. What can we do?

As parents, it's up to all of us to ensure that our kids, especially our out-of-shape, over-fat kids, are getting the proper physical activity that will rev up their fat-burning engines by increasing muscle, and force them to breathe deeply and sweat. It's our job as parents to see to it that our sons and daughters get moving. This may mean joining them for a home work-out, finding a gym that has a children's physical activities program (rare) or placing them in an after-school fitness program. Because the whole fitness thing may be new, it may take some creative thinking on our part to make kid fitness work. It takes hard work, dedication and ingenuity to make them feel good about being more physically active. But rest assured, if we do not address our kids' level of physical activity, they are sure to fail to attain their fat-loss goals. Physical activity is an essential part of increasing their cellular activity. Remember: an active cell is a fat-burning cell.

IF YOU FALL DOWN, JUST GET BACK UP AGAIN!

One thing I have noticed with many parents of obese children is that they hesitate to place their child into a structured sport, for fear that their child will fall behind and be ridiculed by the other young athletes. This concern is valid. Organized sports can place great emphasis on winning and less on having fun, participation and fitness. The over-fat child can be at a distinct disadvantage when playing sports such as football, gymnastics, soccer, volleyball, softball, hockey and the like. However, this does not mean that the child is doomed to sit on the bench. Over-fat kids, more than any other children, should be kept on the move. They need to be more physically active than other children because they have more to gain by losing fat and raising their level of fitness. A structured program is still necessary, but over-fat kids should become comfortable with their body and personal fitness before participating in any organized sports. Physical activity must always be fun and productive for them if they are going to get the fat-burning results they're after.

There should be good exercise programs available at their school. If not, it's likely time to create an awareness among the school faculty, as well as the parents of other over-fat kids that there is a need for special physical activities directed toward the over-fat or out-of-shape child. A word of caution is in order however. No child wants to be singled out—not a child with a learning disability, a physical handicap or one with too much fat. A school-based physical activity program for over-fat kids must not look like it's just for the over-fat, otherwise there is a good chance that the other children will make fun of them. We must help to build their self-esteem at the same time we build them physically.

Tony is just 12, but he already is burdened with the responsibility of being alone at home after school until his mom gets home after work at around 5:30. This leaves Tony with about two hours alone

to do his homework, watch TV, and snack on juices, chips and
cookies. Tony likes his snacks, and his excessive body fat shows it,
but what to do?

Tony tried after-school programs, but since he was over-fat, he
just didn't feel like he fit in. And the part of town he lives in is not
as safe as it once was, so playing outside is risky. Tony's parents prefer
that he just come home and lock the door.

Tony's not alone. Tony is one of an estimated 7 million kids in North America who are under the age of 13 and home alone after school. Helping Tony to improve his health and level of fitness requires careful planning. Perhaps families in the neighborhood can band together and form a play group after school, with stay-at-home parents taking turns interacting with the kids, or, when Tony's parents arrive home, maybe the family can join in a group fitness program. The goal is to be creative and physical.

Television viewing after school may have to go. Research shows that the increase in television viewing, video game playing and Internet use by kids has resulted in a rise in childhood obesity. When these leisure activities were cut back and replaced with more physical after-school play like tag, basketball and climbing a jungle gym, the kids who were over-fat lost excess body fat and got healthier. Giving home-alone kids not only the responsibility to be by themselves, but also taking the responsibility for their own health and fitness, will be a big step in the right direction. Parents must first set the example in helping kids see the light at the end of the tunnel, because no one wants to see an over-fat kid become an obese adult.

PART II

Food
for Thought

We all know that the foods we eat play a major role in how much fat we wear, but the question remains, exactly how does food make us fat in the first place? While the foods we consume contain a full array of *micro*nutrients such as vitamins, minerals and enzymes, the bulk of our food consists of what are called the *macro*nutrients: carbohydrates, dietary fats and dietary proteins.

The macronutrients contain the energy (measured in calories, a unit of heat energy) that we use to help build and rebuild our bodies. They also replenish our energy stores, including muscle and liver glycogen (stored sugar), and fat (triglycerides). The carbohydrates and dietary proteins we eat each contain 4 calories per gram, while dietary fats contain about 9 calories per gram. Some foods, such as sirloin steak, which contains a lot of dietary proteins and dietary fats, are obviously more energy dense than a carrot, which contains carbohydrates and a lot of water. We pick and choose among these food options every day. This brings us to what we all know about how we became over-fat in the first place: we choose (and eat) more calories than we can use.

Most of us are born with the capacity to burn fat efficiently, although unfortunately some of us are sluggish from the start. Other people are so ready to burn fat that it doesn't seem to matter what they eat. As we age, depending on how we treat our bodies, we can maintain a powerful system that burns fat and keeps us lean or develop one that runs on sugar and hoards our excess fuel. While genetics do control our fate somewhat, we still have the ability to retrain our bodies to become fat-burning warriors, and good foods at the right times will help to do this. It's not only the *amount* of food that we eat that determines how over-fat we are; the *type* of foods and *when* we eat them count as well.

SIZE MATTERS

While we're on the subject of quantity, remember when a cinnamon roll easily fit into your hand? No more. Today the commercial muffins, cinnamon rolls and sticky buns we find at the typical family restaurant are the size of softballs, with 450 calories each. There is a very close connection between the increase in eating meals away from home and how fat people are getting, and the restaurants are the culprits. In the land of plenty, we've come to expect a lot for our money. No fancy French food for us! We see a small meal come to the table, perfectly presented but definitely modest in size, and we ask ourselves, "Where's the beef?" Today we expect a lot of food, and restaurants have been more than happy to give it to us. Super-size meals for super-size people. But what does "super size" really mean? It means more calories, more insulin and ultimately more body fat. Even at more formal restaurants, we've come to expect plates heaped with pasta, rice, potatoes and breads. And what do we do? We clean our plates.

In a 1999 study of 129 women, those who reported eating out the most consumed on average 280 more calories each day than their dine-in counterparts. That's a lot of extra energy that was likely stored as fat. An interesting experiment set up by CBS Television and the University of Illinois showed the level of gluttony we have become accustomed to. During a movie matinee showing, each patron was given popcorn. In Group One, the moviegoers received a large tub; the patrons in Group Two were each given a super-size tub. The researchers documented that the people who were given the super-size tub consumed 50% more popcorn than those who received the smaller (relatively speaking here) tub. What does this mean? It means that we will eat whatever is placed in front of us, without objection.

Not only do we *not* object to a large size when it's pressed upon us, when our turn comes in the fast-food line, we actually request it! We all want the greatest value for our dollar. We look up at the menu board and say "Make mine super-size." We choose the double-patty hamburger, the super fries and the huge soft drink containing enough calories and high-glycemic foods to rocket our insulin levels to Mars. This brings us to one of the most innocent-looking enemies in the Fat Wars: liquid candy (a k a soda pop).

If we really want to drive lots of calories into our fat cells, then all we've got to do is down a soft drink loaded with sugar, caffeine and phosphorous. Years ago, a soft drink was 236 mL, but no more. Today it's common to see cups holding more than a liter of pure refreshment. But we don't usually count sugar-laden soft drinks as liquid body fat. We count the solid foods we eat, but don't give the liquid candy a second thought. Kids who drink an average of 355 mL of soda a day consume 200 more calories than kids who don't. And since many kids drink pop instead of milk or water (soft drinks outsell milk two to one), there's a good chance that they're drinking a lot more than 355 mL of a beverage that is nutritionally worthless.

Many artificially sweetened drinks make people edgy, either from the sweetener itself, or from the caffeine the drink companies are adding. If you don't think caffeine has an effect on our calorie consumption, think again. Caffeine is added to pop to bring us back for more. Numerous studies have shown that just 100 mg of caffeine a day will cause us to become addicted to pop. (It does cause withdrawal symptoms for a few days when you cut back.) The result is that no one withdraws, they just keep on filling up their super gulps. A 950 mg serving of one of the leading colas contains between 98 and 125 mg of caffeine, enough to get us really hooked. Kids may be at even greater risk because although they weigh less, they can down a big drink as if it were water, producing negative effects such as nervousness, stomachache and nausea. If that wasn't enough of a problem, the phosphates added to various soda pops increase kidney stone formation.

Drink water first, iced tea (decaf if available) or at least go for the small size of pop instead of the bucket size. And stay away from the super-caffeine pops like Mountain Dew® or Surge®, which have over 50 mg of caffeine in 355 mL. It may be tough to break the habit for two to three days, but after that you should be able to break free. Get the pop out of your life and begin the process of losing the fat.

6

Macro-Fuel One:
Carbohydrates

Carbohydrates come mainly from plants and the final products include grains, vegetables, fruits and refined carbohydrates such as flour and sugar. In order for foods to become usable substances in the body, their matter must first be broken down into their simplest forms: molecules. In the case of carbohydrates, they are broken down into simple sugars like glucose—each carbohydrate food has an equivalent expressed as sugar. (For instance, a baked potato has about 50 g of starch, which is the equivalent of about 60 mL of sugar.) Those refined carbohydrates (and sugars) raise blood glucose levels quickly and are the single biggest contributor to those high insulin levels. As we saw in Chapter 2, elevated insulin levels are an over-fat person's nightmare. The body can't access fat as a fuel source as long as there are high levels of insulin floating around. And a very large percentage of people, especially over-fat people, have high resting insulin levels most, if not all, of the time. In fact, not only do over-fat people have high insulin levels in their blood, but the cells have high levels too, and this creates a sluggish metabolism.

The overflow of insulin has been proven to spell the end to fat-loss goals and, in the process, cause a lot of destruction. In a 1996 experiment, people were given substances to increase their insulin levels as well as their blood sugar levels, plus an infusion of various fatty acids. The experiment showed that glucose and insulin determine how effectively fat gets burned as fuel: high glucose/insulin levels reduced the concentration of the enzyme that transports fatty acids for burning to 45% of normal.

The high-carbohydrate diet creates a vicious circle. At the muscle cell level, years of poor diet, likely combined with a lack of exercise, and stress have caused the muscle cells to go flat. Like a stagnant pond that is practically devoid of life, our muscle cells just don't function as they should, so not only is there an oversupply of blood sugar, it can't get into the flat muscle cell; it's floating around in the bloodstream with no place to go. An alarm rings out in the pancreas: pump out more insulin—NOW! For hours, perhaps all day, insulin is elevated to deal with this blood sugar onslaught. As we know, this stops fat burning cold. In fact, it jams a great amount of the meal right into fat cells. You know the saying, "Might as well apply it directly to my hips"? Nothing burned, everything gained.

This high insulin will not be detected by the standard blood sugar tests done for a routine checkup. We won't have high blood sugar levels as long as the pancreas is pumping out lots of insulin. As far as the blood sugar test is concerned, everything is cool—no diabetes here. But high insulin levels cause damage to the cardiovascular system and keep us fat. The reason why 95% of all people with Type 2 diabetes are over-fat is because they have had high insulin levels over a long period of time—their pancreas was pumping it out to combat the excess blood sugar. Eventually the cells went from working poorly with insulin to becoming insulin resistant. The result? Type 2 diabetes.

In the case of people with cardiovascular disease, there is an excellent chance that they have high insulin levels, too, and excess carbohydrate consumption does much more than just raise insulin levels. The fallout from the overindulgence on the wrong kinds of carbs also raises blood triglyceride and cholesterol levels.

SIMPLY COMPLEX

The carbohydrates we eat that get turned into blood sugar much too fast are another enemy in the Fat Wars. For a long time, researchers thought that simple sugars (which are found in fruits, vegetables, milk and milk products) entered the bloodstream faster than any other sugars, but in the 1980s some Australian and Canadian pioneers in the field of carbohydrate and blood sugar research discovered otherwise. Those complex carbohydrates we came to worship as the bastions of health—the breads, potatoes, pasta and rice we consumed as the staples of our diets—were actually raising insulin levels through the roof, even more so than simple carbs.

Today, many carbohydrate-rich foods are ranked according to how fast they get into the bloodstream, on a scale from 0 to 100 called the glycemic index. The index measures the speed at which the carbohydrates break down and put sugar into the bloodstream. Some break down quickly during digestion and raise blood sugar to dangerous levels. These have the highest glycemic index rating. Glucose, at a dose of 50 g, is used as the benchmark and is given a rating of 100 because it raises blood sugar super fast. Other carbohydrates are ranked in relation to glucose.

> ### The Glycemic Index
> The glycemic index, or GI, is a specific ranking of various foods based on their immediate effect on blood glucose (sugar) levels. The GI measures how much your blood glucose increases over a period of two or three hours after a meal.
>
> Dr. David Jenkins, professor of nutrition at the University of Toronto, was the first to develop the concept of the glycemic index to help determine which foods were best suited for people with blood sugar disorders (diabetes). In March 1981 Dr. Jenkins released a groundbreaking study called "Glycemic Index of Foods: A Physiological Basis for Carbohydrate Exchange." In the subsequent 15 years, hundreds of clinical studies in the United Kingdom, France, Italy, Canada and Australia have proved the value of the glycemic index.

To develop a glycemic index rating for a particular carbohydrate, 50 g of the food is consumed, and then the subject's blood sugar level is measured. If the carbohydrate raises blood sugar quickly, it's given a high number on the glycemic index. It is the high-glycemic carbohydrates that we should consume less of because they overstimulate insulin production, which reduces calorie burning (as well as burning out the pancreas and causing heart damage). Low-glycemic carbs can help keep insulin levels low so that more calories can be burned up.

A selected list of carbohydrate foods grouped by their respective glycemic ratings is shown in the *Fat Wars* Glycemic Index on pages 51 and 52. This is a small list, and there are obviously many more foods to consider, but it will give a good indication of which foods to consume and which ones to cut back on (or avoid altogether). Many favorite foods, including some we were told were good diet foods, are actually in the highest group on the glycemic index. Master the glycemic index and you'll be better able to sort enemies from allies in the Fat Wars.

Just because a food has a higher glycemic index rating does not mean that we should avoid it entirely. We can combine a small amount of a high-glycemic food with a quantity of low-glycemic foods and get a balance. Foods like carrots, which have a fairly high rating, are fine in moderation. Remember that a carrot is full of water, and we would have to eat a half dozen carrots to get a significant boost. Calorie-dense carbohydrates like breads, pastas, rice and potatoes must be eaten in moderation. It's important to realize that how a food is cooked will affect its glycemic rating. For example, pasta cooked *al dente*, or harder pasta will take longer to break down than soft pasta. Usually the longer a food is cooked, the more quickly it will break down into sugars.

THE FAT WARS GLYCEMIC INDEX
The following foods are grouped according to their rating on the glycemic index. The best carbohydrate choices are in the low-glycemic group in the index. Restock the refrigerator and pantry to emphasize low-glycemic foods. Ditch the refined breads and breakfast cereals, baked and mashed spuds, white rice, toaster waffles, rice cakes, tator tots and french fries. The consumption of high-glycemic foods raises insulin and reduces glucagon; this prevents the burning of body fat. Any high-glycemic foods should be consumed in the minimum amount and combined with dietary proteins and fats in a meal. The only exception is a high-glycemic drink after exercise. But remember, even a low-glycemic food can make you fat if you eat too much of it.

LOW-GLYCEMIC FOODS: Rated 20–49 (Allies)

• All bran cereals	• Grapefruit	• Plums
• Apples	• Milk	• Soybeans
• Apple juice	• Muesli cereal	• Strawberries
• Barley	• Navy beans	• Wild rice
• Berries	• Oranges	• Yogurt (no added
• Black-eyed peas	• Peaches	sugar)
• Bulgur	• Peanuts	
• Butter beans	• Pears	
• Cherries	• Peas	

**MODERATE-GLYCEMIC FOODS: Rated 50–69
(Double Agents: LIMIT CONSUMPTION)**

• Basmati rice	• Lima beans	• Raisins
• Beets	• Oatmeal	• Sourdough bread
• Buckwheat	• Pasta (soft cooked)	• Sucrose (table
• Carrots	• Peas	sugar)
• Cereal (low sugar)	• Potato chips	• Sweet potato
• Corn on the cob	• Potatoes (red, white)	• Whole wheat bread
• Grapes	• Pumpernickel bread	(100% stone-ground)
• Ice Cream		

HIGH-GLYCEMIC FOODS: Rated 70–100 (EAT AT YOUR OWN RISK)

- Apricots
- Bagels
- Bananas (ripe)
- Breakfast cereals (refined with added sugar)
- Corn chips
- Cornflakes
- Corn syrup solids
- Crackers and crispbread
- Doughnuts
- Glucose and glucose polymers (maltodextrin-based drinks)
- Hamburger and hotdog buns
- Honey
- Jelly beans
- Maltose
- Mango
- Muffins (due to the processed flour)
- Pancakes
- Papaya
- Parsnips
- Puffed rice or wheat
- Potato (baked)
- Rice cakes
- Shredded wheat
- Soft drinks and sport drinks (added sugars)
- Toaster waffles
- Watermelon
- White bread
- White rice
- Whole wheat bread

CHOOSING CARBS THE GLYCEMIC WAY

One trick to keeping blood sugar low, and insulin in check, is to eat like a caveman. That is, eat like we did when all we had access to were natural, unprocessed foods. The foods at the bottom of the food chain, the unprocessed fruits and vegetables that are high in fiber and water, are among the lowest on the glycemic index. In contrast, the highly processed rice, breads and rice cakes—the ones we either "improved" or that are completely artificial—are among the highest.

The worst of the high-glycemic carbs are scattered like land mines all around us in the form of fat-free snacks. Fat-free does not mean calorie-free and, more often than not, it means high glycemic. When in doubt, check the *Fat Wars* Glycemic Index and eat the foods in the first group (with a rating below 50) as much as possible. There are whole books available about the glycemic index that contain big tables with dozens of foods listed. These tables will likely grow in the future as more people become interested in the glycemic index.

While the *Fat Wars* Glycemic Index is very useful when selecting carbohydrate foods, it was never designed to be the only guide to the way we should eat. We should also take into consideration the overall amount of macronutrients we ingest. After all, carbohydrates are not the only thing that can make us fat. Overconsumption of calories in general will also pack on the extra layers. The amount and kinds of fats, dietary proteins, the fiber content and the overall nutritional value of the foods we consume are also of paramount importance. French fries and potato chips have a lower glycemic rating than a baked potato, but that doesn't make them a great food choice because of the type of dietary fats they contain. (A slice of cardboard has a low glycemic rating, but this isn't a good reason to eat it either.)

Carbohydrates can play a key role in health and burning body fat, provided they are low glycemic, fresh and unprocessed as much as possible, and packed with phytonutrients and fiber. Research shows that when a high-carbohydrate diet is replaced with one containing more protein, the benefits include lower blood fats, reduced insulin and an increase in fat burning. Make your meals rich in fresh vegetables and fruits, lean meats and other dietary proteins, and low in grains and processed cereals.

Low-Glycemic Facts
- Low-glycemic foods do not stimulate food-craving hormones.
- Low-glycemic food plans are not based on starvation or deprivation.
- Low-glycemic food plans have been proven to reduce the incidence of Type 2 diabetes and to help control Type 1 and Type 2 diabetes, hypoglycemia and hypertension.
- High-glycemic foods elevate insulin and blood glucose, stimulate fat-storage, exacerbate hyperactivity and reduce sports performance. Low-glycemic foods do not.

7

Macro-Fuel Two:
Dietary Fats

Dietary fats (fatty acids) don't always make us fat. Over the last twenty years, we have seen low-fat diets hit the market in a big way, leading us to believe that if we replaced fat-laden foods with low-fat carbohydrates, our problems would be solved. Because dietary fat has 9 calories per gram, compared to carbohydrate's 4 calories, we assumed that if we just reduced our consumption of dietary fats and raised our consumption of carbohydrates, we would lose fat. As we know, over the last decade, we've become even fatter, with nearly 30% more of us moving into the obese category. Too many high-glycemic carbs are not the answer to our fat-burning woes. Elimination of dietary fats is not the answer either. Dietary fats are broken down into individual fatty acids and glycerides. Fat consumption is okay—it's just that the wrong type of dietary fats can turn muscle cells into lousy fat burners. Many research studies show that if we keep our dietary fat consumption within the range of 20–35% of total food intake, it will not make us fat.

Genetically we haven't changed much from thousands of years ago when we consumed wild game, fish and nuts. How were these foods different from the foods of today? Not only were they low-glycemic, they contained good amounts of friendly fats. Today, our diets have a totally different dietary fat content than the ones we were genetically made for, which is why we suffer from many "unfriendly fat"-related diseases, including cardiovascular disease, arthritis, diabetes, hypertension and obesity.

SEPARATING THE ALLIES FROM THE ENEMIES

Dietary fats are necessary in our diets, but it's the type of fat that we eat that can make all the difference in the world. Natural whole foods contain dietary fats as part of their structural components, and have a balance of saturated fats, monounsaturated fats and polyunsaturated fats. The wrong fats, like trans fats or too much saturated fat from animal products, can cause our fat-burning muscle cells to become sluggish and lazy. As long as we don't overdo our consumption of dietary fats, and we eat the right kind, we can gather allies in the Fat Wars.

Each of the different dietary fats has a particular chemical composition. Specifically, each is made up of a chain of carbon atoms, with hydrogen atoms attached. The type of dietary fat (and how it works with the rest of the body's chemistry) is determined by the length of the carbon chain, as well as the number and arrangement of the hydrogen atoms that are attached.

We have all heard the terms saturated and unsaturated fat before, but how many of us really understand the difference?

Saturated Fat: A saturated fat is simply a dietary fat with no vacancies. This means that the carbon chain is carrying its maximum number of hydrogen atoms. These fats are vital to our biochemistry, but our bodies can usually manufacture all that they need from raw materials (food). Saturated fats have a molecular straight structure that allows them easy access into our already bulging fat cells. In essence, they are only useful as fuel, and no one has to remind us of how much extra fuel we are already carrying. They are found in high concentrations in meat and dairy products. In excess, they contribute to obesity, cardiovascular disease, certain cancers and insulin insensitivity. By limiting consumption of saturated fats, we'll improve muscle cell activity, increase their fat-burning rate and reduce the deposit of fatty acids. (High saturated fat combined with low-fiber diets are even worse; they are associated with high insulin levels leading to over-fatness, obesity and prediabetic conditions.)

Unsaturated Fats: An unsaturated fat is a dietary fat with vacancies on its carbon chain. A monounsaturated fat has a single, special bond between the two carbon atoms without hydrogen partners; a polyunsaturated fat has more vacancies (and more carbon bonds). It is the various vacancies along the carbon chain that give the various fats their special roles. The more vacancies the carbon chain has, the more biologically active the dietary fat can be, and the more biological places it can go besides the fat cell.

Monounsaturated fats (MUFA) are important to overall health, especially when the goal is low blood triglyceride, LDL cholesterol and glucose levels. A high consumption of MUFA contributes to a lower incidence of cardiovascular disease and diabetes. MUFAs also act as antioxidants, reducing the free radicals produced by LDL cholesterol oxidation. Research on people with diabetes has shown that a diet high in MUFA can reduce blood levels of triglycerides by 19%, LDL cholesterol by 14% and V(ery)LDL cholesterol by 22%. That's a sizable decrease considering that many lipid- and cholesterol-lowering drugs don't deliver these kinds of results, and carry with them serious side effects.

Oils rich in MUFAs include olive, canola and high-oleic safflower oil. They're a great addition to our arsenal of fat-fighting weapons. (Mediterranean diets are high in MUFAs because of the high amount of olive oil consumed. As a matter of fact, Mediterranean people consume up to 40% of their diets as fat and still have some of the lowest incidences of heart disease in the world today.) Just remember: MUFAs are high-calorie dietary fats themselves, so when adding them to foods, take away other calories from harmful fats or high-glycemic carbohydrates.

NOT JUST GOOD FATS—THEY'RE ESSENTIAL!

Linoleic acid (LA), known as omega-6, and alpha-linolenic acid (ALA), known as omega-3, are classed as essential fatty acids (EFAs). These dietary fats are different from other fats because they cannot be manufactured by the body; they must be consumed. They are, of course, polyunsaturated. Omega-6 has four hydrogen vacancies on the chain with two special bonds between carbon pairs; omega-3 has six hydrogen atom vacancies.

These two fats are considered essential because they supply the building blocks of various structures within the body. This includes the cell membranes that enclose every one of our 100 trillion cells and the raw ingredients in the structure of eyes, ears, brain, sex glands and adrenal glands. They also regulate the traffic of substances in and out of our cells, keeping foreign molecules, viruses, yeasts, fungi and bacteria outside of cells, and keeping cell proteins, enzymes, genetic material and organelles (like the mitochondrion where fat is burned) inside the cell. Because EFAs carry a slight negative charge, they repel each other, spreading out in all directions to carry oil-soluble toxins from deep within the body to the skin surface for elimination. EFAs also store electric charges that produce the bioelectric currents important for nerve, muscle and cell membrane functions, and the transmission of messages from the brain.

Without an adequate supply of these friendly fats, our fat-burning potential again comes to a halt. Fat can actually help burn fat? Yes! These essential fats work together to increase the overall amount of oxygen utilized by the cells to produce energy—and the more oxygen we transport to our cells, the faster we burn body fat. EFAs increase the body's metabolic rate and also increase the insulin efficiency of the body. Therefore, by making the omega-6 and omega-3 fatty acids the main sources of dietary fats, we can greatly reduce our unwanted fat stores.

> **The Essentials on Essential Fatty Acids**
> EFAs can:
> - regulate oxygen and energy transport
> - help to form red blood cells
> - keep hormone-producing glands active
> - help make joint lubricants
>
> Both omega-6s and omega-3s are also precursors to hormone-like messengers called prostaglandins, which affect nealy every biochemical process in the body. Prostaglandins from omega-3s are especially important because they:
> - regulate blood pressure, platelet stickiness and kidney function
> - help transport cholesterol
> - help generate electrical currents that make our hearts beat properly
> - build docosahexaenoic acid (DHA), which is needed by the most active tissues—brain, retina in the eyes, adrenal glands and testes
> - help our immune system fight infections
> - help prevent the development of allergies
> - improve insulin sensitivity

The EFAs are not always benign. Overconsumption of omega-6 is linked to an increase in certain cancers and an increase in obesity. When it comes to the maintenance of optimum health and increased fat-burning potential, a partnership between the omega fats is the best medicine with omega-3 being the dominant player. It is the omega-3s that stand out in stimulating fat-burning activity.

Typically in Western industrial nations, human fat cells store more than 50% monounsaturated fatty acids, 30–40% saturated fatty acids and 10–20% polyunsaturates. This is a reflection of the ratio of dietary fats we consume. Among the polyunsaturates in fat-cell triglycerides, the predominant fatty acids are the omega-6s; the omega-3s are usually less than 1% of what's there. This means we're very much omega-3 deficient. Since 1850, omega-3 consumption has decreased to one-sixth its traditional (healthy) level, resulting in an omega-6 to omega-3 ratio of 20:1, with an optimum ratio being between 1:1 for the brain and 4:1 for the lean tissues. High levels of omega-6 EFAs as a whole suppress the uptake of omega-3s into tissues. By increasing the amount of omega-3 essential fatty acids in our diet with foods like flaxseed oil and cold-water fish (containing EPA and DHA), we'll be able to reintroduce this important class of nutrients into our cells.

FINDING FATS AND STORING THEM

The most common oils are extracted from seeds (canola, flax, safflower, sesame, sunflower); grains (corn, wheat germ); fruits (avocado, olive); beans (soy); and nuts (almond, coconut, palm kernel, peanuts, walnut). The molecules in saturated fats are shaped like a straight line and are easily stacked together in a solid mass. These dense fatty acids are very stable; they resist damage from air, light and heat. Saturated fats are found in butter and coconut oil.

Monounsaturated fats (high in oleic fatty acids) are less stable than saturated fats, but more stable than polyunsaturates. When refrigerated they become thick, but at room temperature they become thin again. They are a wise choice when using oil for cooking purposes, but they should never be placed on high heat. Monounsaturated rich oils include olive and canola.

Polyunsaturated fats are the least stable. Safflower and corn oils are the most popular polyunsaturated oils and require careful handling to ensure freshness. The super-polyunsaturated oils are the most rare and are rich sources of essential fatty acids. They are also the least stable. They are found in cold-water fish and oils from flaxseed and, to a lesser extent, in canola and hempseed oil (omega-3s) and in omega-6 seeds such as black currant, borage, evening primrose, safflower, sunflower, corn and flaxseed oil. Oils like cold-pressed flaxseed oil and others are very sensitive to light, air and high temperatures. These oils degrade very quickly and should be refrigerated (or frozen) and kept in a lightproof, tightly sealed container. (Flaxseed oil sold in health food stores is packaged in an opaque bottle—or should be—and is likely refrigerated.) Unrefined oils like sesame and peanut oils are also very active and should not be used for cooking—they should not be exposed to high temperatures. Add them to salad dressings or other non-heated foods for the best results.

A WORD ABOUT UNNATURAL FATS

Frankenstein fats is just another name for artificially altered fats called trans fats. Trans fats include those found in fried foods, margarine and many bakery products. Trans fats have been chemically transformed through heat and hydrogenation (the process of filling in vacancies on the carbon chain by adding hydrogen atoms). By adding hydrogen atoms and altering the structures of healthy cis-essential fats, we give these fats longer shelf lives. Good for business, bad for health. By hydrogenating these once healthy, biologically active fat-keys, we alter them in such a way that they become even more easily incorporated into our cellular membranes. This quirk in our biochemistry causes much confusion at the cellular level leading to a leaking effect in our cellular membrances and ultimately causing chaos with many biochemical functions including the closing down of our fat-burning machinery.

HOW MUCH DIETARY FAT IS ENOUGH?

Just how much dietary fat should a person consume, and what is the ideal ratio of the various fatty acids for maximum fat burning and optimum health? Some people do better on more fats than others, but in general, it's the *type* of fat that's important for improving the metabolic rate and allowing muscle cells to function at their full fat-burning and carbohydrate-storing potential.

Limiting the trans fats, saturated fat and even the omega-6 fatty acid linoleic acid is a good start. I recommend that approximately 30% of calories come from dietary fats—mostly essential fats. Use the recommendations in Chapter 14 to calculate your own requirements for daily fat intake.

8

Macro-Fuel Three:
Dietary Proteins

Dietary proteins play a key role in health and fitness, but I want to make it clear (again) that a balance of carbohydrates, dietary fats and high-quality dietary proteins is the answer when it comes to the overall success with fat loss. Many people never reach their fat-loss goals because of an all-or-nothing approach to their diets. Research has overwhelmingly confirmed that if we consume a proper balance of foods while lowering our overall consumption of high-glycemic, insulin-spiking carbs, we will burn fat.

Most of the high-protein diets we see on the market are really low-carbohydrate diets in disguise. As we have seen, many carbohydrates cause us to gain unwanted fat, but removing them altogether from the diet is not going to solve the problem. To turn the tide, many researchers now recommend scaling back on (but not eliminating) the carbs and increasing the dietary proteins. But why are dietary proteins so important?

The importance of dietary proteins has been documented since the beginning of time. The originators of modern medicine, the Greeks, first named it *Protos*, which means to come first, or of the first rank. Every day our bodies build and rebuild close to 300 billion cells with the raw materials found in dietary proteins. Carbohydrates and dietary fats can supply energy for building these body proteins, but they don't supply the actual raw building materials. Only dietary proteins can do that.

The proteins we get from our foods are made up of amino acids; the digestive process breaks them down into individual amino acids and combinations of amino acids called peptides. They are the building blocks for our organs, muscle cells, transport proteins and enzymes. Dietary proteins are absolutely essential for life and fat-burning success.

We are not only what *we* eat, we are also what our ancestors ate. And guess what? Our ancestors ate lots of dietary proteins. As Dr. Boyd Eaton (see Chapter 2) has pointed out, our early diet consisted of at least 30% protein. Of course the protein our ancestors ate was a little different from much of the protein we consume today. Early humans consumed protein from lean game meats that also contained the essential fatty acids we are often lacking in our diets today. Other research indicates that we were predominantly hunters and then gatherers, but our ancestors had the same genes we have today. Our early ancestors were in some ways much healthier than the high-carbohydrate-loving, grain-fed humans of the agricultural revolution.

PROTEIN VS CARBS

Protein helps elevate our resting metabolic rate throughout the day and night—yes, burn more calories even while we sleep! Compared with a high-carbohydrate meal, the thermic (fat-burning) response from a high-protein meal can be 40% greater, and that's a lot of heat. Research also shows that protein meals increase oxygen consumption by two to three times the rate that comes from a high-carbohydrate meal; this also indicates a much greater increase in the metabolic rate. (Thus, protein consumed with every meal will increase our level of alertness, while high-carbohydrate meals have the opposite effect, leaving us feeling dull and sleepy.) If we don't get enough dietary protein from the foods we eat, we'll slow our metabolism down to a snail's pace.

Research also shows that a diet rich in proteins contributes to greater gains in muscle during resistance training than a high-carbohydrate diet does. Higher-protein meals are also more satisfying, filling us up better than a high-carbohydrate meal and decreasing hunger. Good sources of lean protein include chicken, fish, eggs (preferably egg whites), lean meat (tenderloin cuts), fermented soy (tofu, miso or tempeh), and, of course, high-quality protein isolates from whey and soy. Some newer dietary protein formulas that are very effective at curbing the appetite are the ones containing the AlphaPure® trademark. One of the most important things you can do on the Fat Wars plan is to consume high-quality dietary protein with every single meal.

ALL DIETARY PROTEINS ARE NOT CREATED EQUAL

The actual value of the various dietary protein foods is measured in the Net Protein Utilization Index (NPU), which reflects the biological value, expressed as a percentage of digestibility of a specific dietary protein. The biological value of dietary protein is the efficiency with which that protein deposits the proper proportions and amounts of the essential amino acids needed for anabolism (the building of body proteins). The important factor is not the amount of dietary protein consumed, but the amount of dietary protein that is available to the body after ingestion.

Our bodies all have their own specific amino acid profile, and there is no one food that fits that profile exactly. Other than the dietary protein found in our own mother's milk (perfect protein), all other proteins are rated in the NPU against the next best thing, an egg. The only food to have a higher NPU than whole eggs is whey protein, but since this is an engineered food of sorts, the egg remains the benchmark.

The Net Protein Utilization Index
The foods ranked highest to the lowest NPU are:

PROTEIN	BV (biological value, i.e., % digestible)
High alpha (Alphapure®)	159
Whey protein isolates	110-159
Whey protein concentrate (lactalbumin)	104
Whole eggs	100
Cows' milk	91
Egg whites (egg albumin)	88
Fish	83
Beef	80
Chicken	79
Caseinate and milk protein isolates	77
Soy	74
Rice	59
Wheat	54
Seeds, nuts, legumes (beans), sea vegetables (spirulina and chloriella)	49

Plant-based dietary proteins, aside from non-GMO soy protein isolates, are very low on the list. Active vegans, who only consume 100% plant-based foods, are going to have one heck of a time building and repairing muscle tissue. Many studies have shown that when an athlete's essential dietary protein supply comes exclusively from plant-based protein, that athlete will begin to lose quality muscle and strength almost immediately.

Not only are many vegetable proteins not very high-quality sources of amino acids to begin with, many of these foods (like beans, peas and corn) are loaded with carbohydrates. In addition, a sizable portion of dietary proteins from vegetables is never absorbed because the fiber in these foods binds to the protein. (The only exception to low NPU ratings when it comes to vegetable proteins is soy.)

Most of the dietary proteins we eat should come from foods such as lean cuts of red meat (beef, lamb), white meats (skinless poultry, fish), low-fat dairy products and eggs. Many high-quality animal proteins these days (mainly beef, pork, chicken and eggs) must be prepared carefully to avoid a host of infectious bacteria, including salmonella and E. coli. Animal protein can also be riddled with fat, so choose lean varieties. Fish remains an excellent source of amino acids and essential fatty acids. No matter what the source, be a smart consumer. Buy foods that are as fresh, organic and free run as possible.

Additional dietary proteins should come from supplements of only the highest quality protein powders containing whey isolates, soy isolates, or whey and soy blends. (See Appendix II for some recommendations.)

THE BETTER WHEY

Whey is a by-product of cheese-making. (Whey was actually regarded as waste until scientists researched the profiles of its chemical protein structure, and decided to try and extract that protein.) Early whey protein products were referred to as whey concentrates. They contained as little as 30–40% dietary proteins and were filled instead with huge amounts of fat, lactose (milk sugar) and denatured (damaged) proteins. (A good example of denaturation is what happens to the white of a raw egg when it is cooked. When raw, the egg white can be dissolved in water, but after it is cooked, the protein in the egg white becomes hard and insoluble.) The majority of the products available today come from the newer processes—ion-exchange and cross-flow membrane extraction. They have a higher percentage of dietary proteins than their predecessors—high enough to merit the label "isolates."

The newest generation of whey isolates can contain more than 90% pure dietary proteins with almost no dietary fats and minimal levels of lactose. (They are also very expensive to produce. Due to the increased cost of the newer isolates, many manufacturers tend to mix the isolates with less expensive concentrates and still call them isolates.) There is only a very small percentage of companies using 100% isolates. Since whey protein isolates are the highest quality dietary proteins known to modern science, it's important to read the label.

These proteins are extremely anabolic and are able to increase protein synthesis faster and better than other dietary proteins. Their superior amino acid profile gives them the edge over other dietary proteins when it comes to their digestibility and incorporation into muscle tissue.

The most exciting potential of whey protein isolates is their ability to increase our immune response—particularly in the fight with cancer. The protein also aids in fat burning and muscle growth, works as an appetite depressant and can be used by those who are lactose intolerant.

NON-GMO SOY ISOLATES

More and more research is popping up to substantiate the many benefits of soy protein isolates. Soy protein isolates closely meet human needs when it comes to the supply of valuable amino acids. A specific brand of soy isolates called Supro® is equivalent to the egg when it comes to protein quality. (See Appendix II for more information.)

Soy isolates are high in the branched chain amino acids (BCAAs) needed for muscle energy and growth, and high in arginine, which is needed to stimulate anabolic hormones like human growth hormone (HGH). It is also high in the most abundant amino acid in muscle tissue, glutamine (containing twice the levels of whey). Glutamine is another amino acid that drives anabolic metabolism.

Soy protein isolates have the ability to reduce harmful free radicals, build quality muscle, help speed metabolism (through thyroid output), increase growth hormone levels and supply valuable bioavailable calcium, folic acid and iron.

Another incredible effect of soy is its ability to lower bad cholesterol and increase good cholesterol levels. Soy protein does this so well in fact, that as of October 26, 1999, the U.S. Food and Drug Administration approved the use of health claims regarding the role of soy protein in reducing heart disease.

The normal range for cholesterol in a healthy human being should be around 160 mg/dl of blood. The risk of cardiovascular disease starts to rise at cholesterol levels exceeding 200 mg/dl. Over 100,000,000 North Americans have blood cholesterol levels over 200 mg/dl. That's almost half the North American population. Still more and more people are being measured with blood cholesterol levels over 240 mg/dl; that's almost a sure ticket to Heart Attack Alley.

Body fat levels have nothing to do with cholesterol levels, so being extra lean doesn't mean there's no chance of having high levels of cholesterol. Cholesterol is only contained in foods from animal sources, and recent evidence uncovered by The Colgan Institute of Nutritional Science states that it is not the dietary fat content in these foods, but the dietary protein itself that raises cholesterol levels.

The amino acid structure of dietary proteins also has a direct effect on hormones. Levels of the antiaging, fat-reducing, human growth hormone have been increased by using amino acids like L-arginine and ornithine alpha-ketoglutarate. Animal proteins usually contain high levels of L-lysine and much lower levels of L-arginine. High levels of L-lysine have been shown to work in opposition to L-arginine, which can affect the amount of HGH that is released. High levels of L-lysine can in fact increase the production of insulin by reducing the amount of glucagon, making it very difficult to lose body fat. This change in the ratio of insulin to glucagon signals the liver to make large amounts of fat and cholesterol.

As noted in the section on women and menopause, scientists have known for years that Asian people have a much lower incidence of blood cholesterol and certain types of cancers. The relative absence of these diseases has been linked to their high consumption of plant foods, mainly soy. Soy protein has a much more favorable arginine-to-lysine ratio, which increases glucagon levels, facilitates the fat-burning effect and lowers cholesterol levels. In summary, the benefits of soy protein include (but are not limited to) effective lowering of insulin-to-glucagon ratio; supply of cancer-fighting, immune-boosting phytochemicals/isoflavones; increase in bone density of postmenopausal women; and improvement in kidney function.

HOW MUCH DIETARY PROTEIN?

According to the Recommended Dietary Allowances (RDA) set out in the U.S. for dietary proteins, we shouldn't be taking in any more than 0.8 g of protein per kilogram of body weight. While this amount may be acceptable for people who never move, many researchers (including myself) believe that it is much too low for someone who wishes to gain muscle. There is actually a statement in the U.S. *RDA Handbook* that reads, "In view of the margin of safety in the RDA no increment is added for work or training." Apparently these experts are under the impression that nobody in North America works, let alone works out.

This certainly does not mean that we should overconsume dietary proteins at any one sitting—too much protein in one meal can stress the liver and kidneys. The upper limit, depending on body size and activity level, seems to be 30–40 g at one sitting.

We are all biochemically different and therefore our dietary protein requirements are different as well. Just assume that the more active you are, the more dietary protein you will need to repair the body. Dr. Lee Coyne points out in his book, *Fat Won't Make You Fat,* that according to some of the most respected researchers in the field of nutrition, the RDAs for dietary proteins can be too low by at least a factor of three. This assumption is further backed by research by Dr. Emanuel Cheraskin, formerly from the University of Alabama. After assessing the Cornell Medical Index Health Questionnaire filled out by 1,040 dentists and their spouses, Dr. Cheraskin found that those who consumed two to three times the RDA of dietary proteins had the fewest medical health problems.

Individual dietary protein intake and absorption are also affected by the way the proteins are prepared (raw, cooked) as well as the accessory nutrients that are available for the assimilation of the proteins. Dietary proteins require a full array of the B vitamins in order to be properly utilized and incorporated into body tissues.

One of the most effective ways to increase fat-burning potential is to increase anabolic metabolism (anabolism), the rebuild and repair process of the body. This is the rate at which we are able to turn over new cells and repair our bodies. Dietary proteins are the driving force behind anabolism due to their ability to supply the nitrogen necessary for repair.

We are very complex structures of nearly 100 trillion cells. These cells are constantly regenerating as our bodies replace our entire muscular system approximately every six months. Therefore, the nutrients we feed ourselves today will determine who and what we become tomorrow. The quality of dietary proteins we consume is of the highest priority. To help with protein requirements, I highly recommend protein shakes so I've included sample recipes at the end of Chapter 11. These liquid protein meals may just give your fat-burning team the upper hand in the Fat Wars.

The importance of consuming only the highest quality dietary protein sources can never be taken for granted. Since we are constantly renewing the molecules of our structure every second of every day, we have to be accountable for what we put in our mouths, and what ultimately becomes part of our structure. We recognize that we must all respect the ecosystem on earth so that we may breathe the air of the future. The human body is also an ecosystem just as complex and beautiful as the world we live in, and it too demands respect. If we think twice about littering on this planet, why not think twice about littering in our own bodies?

I think the sports nutrition researcher, Dr. Michael Colgan, said it best when he wrote, "Oh, the human system is ingenious at making do with inadequate building materials, patching, stitching and pinch-hitting, but it can't build premium tissue from garbage. A Twinkies-and-coffee diet produces a Twinkies-and-coffee body. For optimum performance you have to eat optimum protein to build optimum structure—period."

9

Constant Craving

Janice pulled her hand out of the cookie bag. Both were empty. Of course they were. It had taken her less than 10 minutes to scarf down the dozen or so White Chocolate Macadamia Nut Sensations. She felt a twinge of guilt as her tongue corralled a wayward crumb on her upper lip and swept it into her mouth.

So much for that diet. She'd lasted a whole seven days this time. Last time the cravings got to her before the end of the third day. But then again, that wasn't totally her fault: losing her job and having her car towed on the same day were more than any dieter should be expected to deal with. Besides, that tub of Triple Mocha Almond Fudge Surprise was not only much cheaper than a prescription for Prozac, it was—she rationalized—healthier for her in the long run. At least she'd been smart enough to buy the brand with 100% real cream; as a woman approaching her forties, she knew she was at risk of developing osteoporosis and needed to build up her calcium intake.

This time, she wouldn't be so hard on herself. At least she was staying away from the cigarettes. So what if she put on a few pounds? She was saving her lungs from further damage. And winter clothing was so accommodating, really. If she wore enough layers on top of her skin, no one would ever notice the extra rolls forming beneath it.

This is how the Fat Wars are slowly but surely lost as we set ourselves up for defeat by our own chemistry and fat deposits grow throughout our bodies, despite our best intentions. In "Her Fat," I touched on why women crave extra calories as they age and their estrogen levels drop. I talked about the neurotransmitter, serotonin, and its role in regulating appetite and mood. In this chapter I'll take a closer look at this brain chemical, and discuss why it plays such a large part in everybody's eating habits.

IS EVERYBODY HAPPY?

Serotonin is one of the body's neurotransmitters, a chemical that transfers messages from one nerve cell to another, or from a nerve cell to a muscle cell. Think of our neurons as branches of a tree. As one branch extends, it sends a number of "twigs" off in various directions, reaching toward, but not connecting with, the twigs from another branch. The communication between these twigs (telling the hand to grasp that cookie, for example) is a result of messages being passed back and forth via the neurotransmitters. Studies have shown that different neurotransmitters affect different areas; serotonin has been shown to affect a wide variety of functions, including comprehension and memory, mood, temperature, aggression and appetite.

Our bodies function on a feedback system: when a level of a component is too low, a message is sent out to increase it, or find some way to balance the load. So it is with serotonin. If the amount of available serotonin is low for some reason, the body's feedback system springs into action to ask for a speed-up in the production line. And, being human, our bodies look for the easiest and most direct way to bring the level of serotonin back up to what is necessary. The body craves carbohydrates when serotonin levels are low, and we all know that junk food is filled with carbohydrates.

How Does Serotonin Work?

In the 1990s, Richard and Judith Wurtman, researchers from the Massachusetts Institute of Technology, began to suspect there was a link between low serotonin levels and eating disorders. Richard Wurtman had done studies in the 1970s with research student John Fernstrom that involved tryptophan, an amino acid (a building block of protein) and a precursor of serotonin. (The body can't make serotonin without tryptophan's help with niacin (vitamin B3).) They found that tryptophan rapidly entered the brains of rats that were fed a carbohydrate-rich diet (mostly starch and sugar), enabling the rapid production of serotonin. When they altered the rats' diets to include a protein component, the serotonin levels did not increase, nor was there increased activity in the systems which use serotonin. Eventually they, and other researchers studying tryptophan, found that dietary proteins *prevent* tryptophan from entering the brain. In fact, tryptophan, which occurs in smaller amounts than all the other amino acids in protein, was actually "bullied" out of the way as it competed for passage into the brain.

Where do carbohydrates come in? They don't usually contain trypto-phan; only protein-based foods (and some exceptions like bananas and pineapples) do. So how does eating carbohydrate-rich food increase our brain levels of tryptophan, which increases the production of serotonin? The answer lies in remembering that our body is made up of several systems (skeletal, muscular, hormonal) working together to maintain a balance. When we eat carbohydrates, our digestive system breaks down the carbs into glucose, which can be transported in the bloodstream. Glucose in the blood stimulates the pancreas to release insulin, which escorts the glucose into the cells where it becomes a source of energy. Amino acids are con-stantly surfing the bloodstream, so they get escorted into the cells as well. Remember how I said that tryptophan, in the presence of proteins, gets bullied out of position when it's trying to get into the brain? Well, as it's pushing the other amino acids into the cells, the insulin is giving tryptophan a chance to get into the brain uncontested. If it weren't for the fact that increased insulin interferes with fat burning, we could call this situation a truce: the cells have their energy-producing glucose and amino acids for growth and repair, and the brain has its tryptophan, from which it can produce serotonin on an as-needed basis.

CRAVING CARBS

When you realize how often the body calls on its stores of serotonin —to help with sleep regulation, depression, anxiety, aggression, appetite, temperature regulation, pain sensation and sexual behavior, to name a few—it's no wonder we can run low on serotonin at times. A low level of serotonin could be the result of either a depletion of the stores (through poor dietary habits and high stress, for example), or a decrease in the production (i.e., not enough tryptophan to produce serotonin). In the first case, both internal and external stressors have been implicated, includ-ing premenstrual syndrome, seasonal affective disorder, excessive stress and addictions.

Hippocrates, the father of modern medicine, talked of the healing power of food. His motto was, "Let food be your medicine, and medicine your food." In other words, when life got him down, he, too, probably would have reached for the ice cream if it had been available. But why? Moreover, if we are eating to counteract a low level of serotonin, why do we end up gaining weight? Because regardless of whether we choose starch or sweets, it all gets reduced to glucose, initiating the insulin cycle. The prob-lem is that it takes some time for serotonin to kick in and we keep eating until it does. Besides, all of these carbohydrate-rich foods taste so good, we don't want to stop when we should.

Finally, in our efforts to battle fat, we decide to cut all carbohydrate-rich foods from our diet. Actually, it would work if what we were cutting out was just the sweets and deep-fried snacks, but, unfortunately, cutting out all carbohydrates will have a reverse effect. In fact, the fewer carbohydrates in our diet, the more our bodies crave them (to get the serotonin levels back up). A diet in which we eliminate carbohydrates almost completely may help us lose a few pounds at the beginning, but most of the weight we lose is in water, because each carb molecule is able to hold three or four molecules of water. Also, these very low-carb diets will reduce our serotonin levels, so our bodies will send us on a binge when we go off carbohydrates. (You always hate yourself when this happens—give yourself a break and eat less-processed carbs in moderation.)

What's more, our emotional state also plays a role here. Ever notice that when you're upset, your craving for carbohydrates goes through the roof? This is the body's way of telling us to pump up the serotonin, which is theoretically helping us deal with the emotional stress we're going through. The only problem is that there will soon be more stress from the extra rolls of fat we'll add due to the extra carbohydrates. Nevertheless, oblivious to the future turmoil we are about to create, we reach for the carbohydrates. Remember Janice at the beginning of the chapter? She found the White Chocolate Macadamia Nut Sensations and Triple Mocha Almond Fudge Surprise were quick, easy carbohydrates—just what her body ordered.

We all have our own addictions when it comes to satisfying our cravings. If the sweets aren't what you're looking for, you're probably guilty of going for the savory: chips and dip, perhaps, or a five-topping pizza? Yes, these foods do contain a sufficient supply of carbohydrates that will eventually make their way into our systems. The necessary biochemical conversions will take place, ultimately raising serotonin and supplying us with a great big sigh of relief. But the underlying problem with these food choices is that they will also deposit extra saturated fat into all our eager little fat cells.

These "forbidden" foods are manufactured solely for profit's sake and without a care for our health. Don't think for one minute that the heads of these junk-food corporations go to bed each night thinking about how many people they've helped. They go to bed thinking about how much money they've made—at our expense, literally! The better these foods taste, the more of them we will devour and the greater their profits. And the more dietary fats these foods contain (especially animal fats—the worst kind for our bodies), the better they taste. When we are feeling down, we reach for these comfort foods, which satisfy us for the moment. After all, what can be more special than a devilishly delicious dessert? Aren't we worth it? Of course we are!

GALANIN

If the body is craving something, doesn't that mean it's needed? And shouldn't we give our body what it needs? Ah ha! Let's consider the difference between need and want. When we satisfy a carbohydrate craving (the need part) with fat-laden foods, that enhanced calmness (resulting from the increase in serotonin production) is quickly overshadowed by a feeling of lethargy. The more carbohydrate-rich, fat-laden food we eat—because it tastes so great (the want part)—the more weight we gain and the more lethargic we feel. We are now officially part of the vicious carb circle—but now we're not only depressed again, we're fatter too! We're on our way to becoming overweight, depressed slugs.

What's going on? The answer, identified by Dr. Sara Leibowitz, a professor at Rockefeller University, lies in the effect of a powerful neurochemical called galanin. This chemical is released once a certain amount of dietary fat has entered the body. Galanin competes with serotonin and quickly overpowers it, causing us to feel passive and tired, and interferes with our ability to think. Oh, great! Now we're overweight, depressed and *confused* slugs.

SEROTONIN'S PARTNER—BETTER THAN A LULLABY

Do you remember Mom's remedy for insomnia? A cup of hot milk and a banana. How could Mom know that these tryptophan-rich foods play a part in our sleep cycle? She probably didn't. She was just doing what her mother did for her. But what they have both been doing, in fact, is helping the body as it follows its own circadian rhythm—the natural sleep/wake cycle. Part of that cycle involves melatonin, which is produced as serotonin is depleted. That is, as our daily amount of serotonin is decreased, production of melatonin is increased. The mood-enhancing chemical makes way for the mood-lowering chemical. And since both rely on the precursor tryptophan to ensure the body has adequate levels, it would be wise to consume a diet that has a sufficient supply of tryptophan.

Melatonin

At nighttime, serotonin is converted into our body's sleep regulator, the hormone melatonin. This conversion is controlled by an enzyme called N-acetyl-transferase (NAT), which converts serotonin into N-acetyl-serotonin before becoming melatonin. The reason we don't produce melatonin during the daytime is because the activity of the NAT enzyme is slowed dramatically by daylight hours and intense light (electric or sun).

MAINTAINING TRYPTOPHAN NATURALLY

How do we keep ourselves supplied with tryptophan so serotonin and melatonin can keep us ticking along? Tryptophan, the amino acid needed to manufacture serotonin, can be found in certain foods, including milk and milk by-products, bananas, pineapples, chicken, turkey and high alpha whey protein (Alphapure™). A double-blind, placebo-controlled study (the most respected of studies in the medical community), reported in the prestigious *American Journal of Clinical Nutrition* in June 2000, indicated that whey protein containing high alpha lactalbumin levels (Alphapure™; see Appendix II) could greatly increase (48%>) plasma tryptophan levels in highly stressed individuals. The study also indicated a decrease in stress hormones and a reduced depressive state through the alteration of brain serotonin levels.

Since the U.S. Food and Drug Administration banned the sale of L-tryptophan as an amino acid supplement in 1989, the market has been forced to replace it with expensive prescription drugs. There are some natural alternatives as precursors, such as 5-hydroxy-tryptophan, or 5-HTP as it is referred to in the health field, but it is always recommended to try the natural food approach first to top up your tryptophan levels.

10

Starving

How many times have we been here and done this? One month has passed since the start of our latest diet, and we're finally ready to face the scale. For 30 days we've painstakingly cut the fat from every morsel of beef, peeled the skin off every breast of chicken and opened our share of tuna cans. If someone were to ask how many calories are in a baked potato or a shrimp salad, we could snap back the answer with the speed of a winning contestant on "Jeopardy." Cutting calories has left us feeling spacey at times, but we hope this time that it's all been worth it.

Stripped and ready to face the dial, we carefully shift our weight onto the scale. At first we cover our eyes. After all, fat is frightening. As we lower our hands from our eyes, we see that the dial reads a number we can actually live with. We've lost 12 lbs. We jump around the room, pumping the air and screaming "12 lbs.!" But the question is: 12 lbs. of what?

We nervously check the full-length mirror. This time things are going to be different. After all, the diet was a success and we've dropped 12 lbs. to prove it. But as we gaze at the reflection, we can see there is some mistake. What we see is not a leaner version of ourselves, but a smaller fat person!

Don't think you're in the minority if you've failed at dieting. Contrary to those weight loss ads we see in magazines and on television, 99% of all diets fail miserably because they fight our genetic makeup. They go against the way the body is designed to work. Don't forget that the body has had centuries of training on the feast/famine cycle and it knows what to do to protect itself. It's not just that diets don't work. Most of them will leave us worse off than if we hadn't dieted at all. Once we finish the diet, not only do the lost pounds reappear, a few more are added for insurance against the next "famine." The more we lose, the more we seem to gain. What's wrong with this picture?

BACK TO FAT BASICS

Remember our 30 billion fat cells? Not only can they expand, they can expand up to 1,000 times their regular size to store fuel as a reserve source of energy. These cells have specific processes (and enzymes) to trigger the storage of fat, and its release. Science is now showing that obesity is usually caused by a dysfunction in one of these two systems. Dieting plays a part here by disrupting the balance of storage and release activity.

The Science of Fat Release and Storage

Science is now showing us that obesity is usually caused by a dysfunction in one of these two systems that deal with fat:

- Lipolytic enzymes are enzymes that are responsible for the *release* of fat from our fat cells. Fat has to be released before it can travel to the fat-burning furnaces in our muscles. One of the most important of these enzymes is hormone-sensitive lipase. The more active this enzyme is, the easier it is for your body to get rid of its fat stores. Lipolytic enzymes are under the direct influence of the hormone glucagon.
- Lipogenic enzymes are enzymes that are responsible for the storage of fat. Once food is broken down through the process of digestion, it is transported to our blood stream where it can either be sent to our muscles to be burned as fuel or sent to our fat cells to be stored as energy for the future. One of the peskiest of these enzymes is lipoprotein lipase. The more active this enzyme is, the fatter you become. Lipogenic enzymes are under the direct influence of insulin.

When you overrestrict your calories, your body begins to produce more of the storage enzyme, lipoprotein lipase. So by starving your body to lose weight, what you are really achieving, along with the loss of muscle tissue, is the production of more fat-storing enzymes to give you even more of what you didn't want in the first place, fat!

Dr. Paul La Chance of Rutgers University analyzed 12 of the most popular diets in 1985 and found that all 12 of them relied on the reduction of calories to the point of serious nutrient deficiency. When we overrestrict our calories by following such diets, our bodies not only suffer from immediate deprivation, they also begin to produce more of the storage enzyme in order to pack away as much as possible, particularly after the period of severe calorie restriction is over. By starving ourselves to lose weight, we're actually setting ourselves up for a fat-storage marathon once the famine is over.

Poll after poll shows that at any given moment, over one-third of women and one-quarter of men are on the latest fad diet. Meanwhile, we know that other studies are showing that North Americans are getting fatter every year. Can you believe that we are spending nearly $40 billion a year on a diet industry that can't deliver results? If you opened a bank account and made weekly deposits, only to find out at the end of the year that you owed the bank money, would you assume it was your fault? Would you say to yourself, "I'll just have to save better next time," and open another account? Of course not, but that's exactly what we do when we go from one failed diet to another.

THE *REALLY* BAD NEWS ABOUT DIETS
Low-calorie diets not only deprive the body of valuable nutrients, they also cause a devastating loss of muscle tissue. "Who cares about muscle? I just want to lose fat!" we say. As we've seen from our quick look at the "generator" and the "furnace," muscle is the prime site for burning fat. The more muscle we carry, the more fat we can burn for energy. Studies show that losing even one ounce of muscle lowers the body's ability to create energy, and reduces our fat burning capacity. When drastic weight loss occurs, this translates into a significant decrease in our resting metabolic rate—all because of this reduction in lean body mass (muscle). The reduced ability to burn fat sets us up for another round of the vicious cycle of fat loss and regain as our "new" body requires even fewer calories to function than it did before.

Not convinced? Consider this:
- 1 lb of muscle can burn up to 70 calories a day
- 70 calories a day equals 490 calories a week or 25,480 calories a year
- There are 3,500 calories in 1 lb of fat. Therefore a lost pound of muscle equals a loss of over 7 lbs of fat-burning capacity annually. If we don't reduce our calorie intake after the diet, those 7 lbs will likely find their way to some of our now-eager-to-store fat cells.

The message is clear: by losing valuable muscle tissue, we are turning down our metabolism, the main engine in the fat-burning process. Every time we diet, we lose some more muscle, lower our metabolism and prime our fat-storing enzymes. We're setting ourselves up for more fat gain, which is exactly what's happening. Since fat is burned within our muscle cells, increasing the amount of muscle tissue, not putting all our energy into cutting calories, is what will ultimately increase the size and efficiency of the fat burners.

Cortisol

The culprit in muscle destruction is in our hormonal systems. Our various hormones regulate many metabolic events in the body. Some of our hormones are anabolic, meaning they help to build body tissues. Testosterone (yes, even for women) and growth hormone come to mind. Other hormones can be considered catabolic, meaning that they stimulate a breakdown of body tissues. The most well-known catabolic hormone is cortisol, a hormone released by the adrenal glands when we are under stress. When we diet—subjecting ourselves to an artificial famine—our bodies consider themselves to be under stress.

When the body recognizes this new stress, it releases a lot of adrenaline and cortisol. These two hormones are responsible for meeting the energy needs of the body in stressful times, and they truly want to help. This is the famous "fight or flight" response we've inherited from our ancestors. Our bodies have developed this incredibly quick up-regulating system to ensure the survival of the human race. By up-regulating our stress hormones, we can quickly break down sugars, dietary fats and dietary proteins into their simplest components in order to supply energy and spare the fat stores. There's no telling how long the crisis will last and stored energy in the form of fat is usually the last to go!

If there isn't a supply of new protein (amino acids) in the system, cortisol will have no other choice but to take it from our body tissues in a process called gluconeogenesis, and muscle tissue is the first to go. Cortisol will steal nitrogen from the structural protein in our muscles. After removing the nitrogen, cortisol rapidly converts the protein to sugar for increased energy and maintenance of blood sugar levels in the brain. This is long-term damage, and a major reason why we gain back weight after a diet. Cortisol eats the muscle that we use to burn fat. Here's an easy equation to remember: excess stress equals excess cortisol, which oftentimes equals fat gain. (And we thought we gained weight during times of high stress because we chowed down so much comfort food. Well, that too.)

As we know, any loss of muscle is a victory for the fat side. Fat wins every time we lose even an ounce of muscle. To spare muscle, we've got to reduce the level of cortisol and/or raise our level of anabolic hormones. We've already mentioned that cortisol is increased during a reduced-calorie diet or fasting. The more calories we deprive ourselves of, the more cortisol is produced. But dieting is not the only way to increase cortisol levels. They're also elevated during many other life stresses—illness, in-law visits, work-induced panic attacks, being caught in a traffic jam, losing a job, losing a loved one or having too many bills to deal with are some others. We're pumping out stress hormones daily, often with no let-up or release. And often we're stressed over anticipated events rather than actual ones. Any way we look at it, stress is stress, whether it's real or imaginary. A famous quote from Mark Twain says it all, "I have been through some terrible things in my life, some of which actually happened." In order to win the war on fat, we have to change our reaction to reality, and learn to face many of the events in our lives with some degree of calm.

The shock method of dieting away the fat just isn't going to work because the body senses this stress and reacts accordingly. When we alter our dietary patterns by going on a low calorie, low-fat, low-protein or low-carb diet, the body picks up on it right away and sends out a stress response. No one fools with nature! And as if that wasn't enough of a problem, by dieting we are also decreasing the production of fat-burning enzymes and increasing fat-storage ones.

TAKE TWO PILLS AND CALL ME WHEN YOU'RE SKINNY!

Scientists have mapped out the key hunger and satiety (fullness) signals that the body uses to modulate appetite and have discovered that they are regulated by a control center in the brain called the adipostat. The adipostat is like the thermostat that regulates the heat in a house. It can signal that we are hungry (I'm famished) or it can signal that we are satisfied (I can't eat another bite!). Dieting, by increasing the stress response (cortisol), puts these signals into turmoil, with the hunger response coming out as the victor.

These hunger signals are so important that major pharmaceutical companies have spent millions of dollars to develop drugs that will control them. Eight new drugs approved by the U.S. FDA work by altering a person's metabolism, signaling the brain to increase the satiety (feeling of fullness) response. The ninth and newest drug called Xenical (Orlistat) prevents absorption of dietary fat from the gastrointestinal tract.

Obesity drugs were never designed for use as a quick fix when it comes to fat loss. Dr. Samuel Klein, M.D., professor of medicine and director of the Center for Human Nutrition at Washington University's School of Medicine, stated in a June 1999 editorial in the *American Journal of Clinical Nutrition* that "drug therapy may be most useful for maintaining rather than achieving weight loss." But still, many over-fat and obese people look to the quickest fix possible, even if side effects come with the deal.

There are no quick fixes when it comes to successful long-term fat loss. Our bodies love fat. They love to store fat, and they hate to give it up. They're like Fat Scrooges. That's why fat loss is such a battle. Developing an understanding of how we can win the war on fat is our best hope, and I will show you how in the following chapters.

Glycomacropeptides (GMPs)

Glycomacropeptides are low molecular weight protein peptides that exert an antibacterial and antimicrobial function on our biochemistry. But it is in their amazing ability to stimulate a hormone that can control our hunger responses that has obesity researchers most excited.

GMPs are powerful stimulators of a hormone called cholecystokinin (CCK), which plays many essential roles in our gastrointestinal system. CCK stimulates the release of enzymes from the pancreas, and increases gall bladder contraction and bowel motility. One of CCK's most incredible actions lies in its ability to regulate our food intake by sending satiation signals to the brains, making it a potential diet aid. In animal studies, a rise in CCK is always followed by a large reduction in food intake. In human studies, whey protein glycomacropeptides were shown to increase CCK production by 415% within 20 minutes after ingestion. On another note, GMPs may also have the ability to prevent indigestion and heartburn. In rat studies, GMPs were able to decrease acid secretion in the stomach by 53%. One can only begin to wonder what other effects we will discover from GMPs in the future.

Not all whey protein isolate contain GMPs. Ion exhange whey protein contains trace amounts or no glycomacropeptide fractions at all. The AlphaPure high alpha whey protein contains up to 20% of this important peptide fractions (see Appendix II).

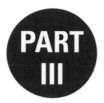

PART III

Let the Change Begin!

> "The greatest discovery of any generation is that human beings can alter their lives by altering their attitudes."
> —Albert Schweitzer

Now it's time to start thinking about how to use your new knowledge to make some changes in your life. In my experience, if you heed the following advice, not only will the fat melt off, it will stay off. Parts I and II of this book have put you in the Know Zone. Now you know how your body works, and understand why previous diets put you on the losing side of the Fat Wars. You also have some idea of what needs to be done to move you beyond your constant battles with body fat.

Now that you have mastered the Know Zone, it's time to move into the Do Zone. You've always had the power to make the right changes, but the difference now is that you know how to make them in a way that makes sense for you.

It's time to choose your strategy, and your strategy will not be the same as anyone else's because you are fighting your own Fat War. Perhaps in the past you were a yo-yo dieter or a binge eater. You may need to conquer your fear of failure because of many failed attempts at permanent fat loss. Rest assured that *Fat Wars* is unlike any weight-loss program you've ever undertaken. Gone are the diets that made you depressed and irritable and drove you back to comfort food. This time, you can lose a considerable amount of fat and gain useful muscle, strength, health and control. By the end of Part III you will be able to take your newfound insights and design your own fat-loss plan. The following chapters will guide you through the eating and exercising principles, and suggest supplements that can help you. I will map out the first 45 days, then give you advice on how to keep seeing results for the rest of your life.

As you read about how to design your own eating and activity plan, resolve to start it today. *Fat Wars* is not another diet book. The synergistic technologies and strategies presented in *Fat Wars* will help you end the war with your body and move on to peace with a lean, healthy one. Is fat loss easy? You already know the answer to that question—of course not. If it was, you wouldn't be having such a tough time and you wouldn't be reading this book. Is permanent fat loss achievable? You bet it is! Fat loss is going to be easier than you ever thought possible by the end of your 45-day transformation period. So what do you say? Let's get started!

11

The Fat Wars
Eating Principles

***Fat Wars* is not intended** to be another "diet" book. I don't want to get into the various dieting strategies for weight loss; instead I want to focus my attention on natural ways to increase the body's ability to burn fat. While this aspect is key, I wouldn't be doing justice to you, the reader, if I didn't discuss daily optimum calorie consumption. It is the combination of effective eating strategies *plus* the types of activity and nutritional supplements discussed in *Fat Wars* that make this plan so effective for overall success.

In order to increase both muscle and your energy levels, and burn fat, you need the proper fuel for your body. Here's an easy equation to remember: energy comes from fuel (measured in calories) and fuel comes from food. This means you must eat, and you must eat regularly. The key is to supply your body with the right fuel at the right intervals. Think of the example of the old clunker and the sports car. A person with a slow metabolism is like the old clunker. The old clunker won't give its owner much performance; as a matter of fact, the owner's happy if the clunker just makes it from point A to point B. The clunker often guzzles gas and doesn't use it efficiently as it chugs along. The person with a slow metabolism usually doesn't use his or her fuel efficiently either—it will be stored as a fuel reserve (body fat). In contrast, a person with sufficient muscle and a fast metabolism is like the sports car. The sports car will give its owner all the performance he or she needs, but it requires the right kind of fuel at the right time to keep performing optimally.

Since metabolism is the speed at which the body processes food into energy, metabolism is the defining factor of body composition. Here's where diets also fail: when we limit the amount of food we take in, our metabolism adjusts by slowing down. (The reverse is also true. If we supply our bodies with sufficient food, our metabolism will adjust by speeding up.)

SNACK YOUR WAY TO GREATER FAT LOSS

When people set out to lose fat, often the first thing they do is to go on a diet. When dieters deprive themselves of nutrition and calories, the first things they cut are snacks, not realizing that the right snacks can play a useful role in winning the war on fat. Dieters who eliminate snacks usually end up eating more at their main meals, quickly packing on the fat. Healthy snacks fill the void between meals when blood sugar dips. Dips in blood sugar, if left unattended, lead to excess calorie consumption at the main meals and possibly binge eating to satisfy cravings.

In order to burn fat the *Fat Wars* way, you should never let more than three waking hours go by without eating something. There is definitely a length of time that is considered too long between meals and, for the most part, it is four hours. At around the four-hour mark, blood sugar levels tend to dip and the body starts to prepare for fat storage by switching into its prehistoric starvation-protection mode. In my own and other researchers' experiences, the ideal length of time between meals is from two and a half to three and a half hours. This way your body never turns on its storage switch.

For most of us, eating every two and a half to three and a half hours will mean between five and six meals per day, but don't get too excited just yet. When I say a meal, I'm not referring to major, calorie-dense meals. I am referring to meals that are between 300 and 500 (no more) calories. This means that they must be calorie sparse yet nutrient dense. This calorie range at each meal has been shown to be optimum for maximum fat-burning potential. Any more than the 500-calorie allotment and the body will store the excess as fat. Of course, I can't overstate the importance of a balance of the macronutrients (carbohydrates, dietary fats and dietary proteins) at each meal with the exception of the last meal, which would exclude the carbohydrate portion—this is imperative for overall success on the *Fat Wars* Plan.

Meal Frequency

The first thing to establish is how often during the day you will be able to eat. This will depend on the maximum amount of time you spend awake. For instance, if you were able to sleep ten hours a night (and not too many people can), you would be awake for 14 hours. Since I am recommending not letting more than two and a half to three and a half hours go by without eating, you should technically be eating at least five meals a day. If you sleep for at least the recommended eight hours a night, you would be awake for 16 hours and would consume five to six meals a day. If you are like the majority of the population, and sleep for approximately six hours a night, then you should consume six meals a day. Each of these meals would stay within the recommended zone of calories and macronutrient profile.

One thing I have learned along the way with various clients is that most people have a hard time with compliance. We are very busy people these days. Whether you are a businessperson, an athlete or a homemaker, preparing (let alone consuming) five to six meals a day can be very arduous. This is one of the reasons I recommend two to three liquid meals per day. As you will see, they are not only lightning fast to prepare, they are also (if prepared properly) nutrient-dense yet calorie-sparse.

Macronutrient Profile

I have done my best to stay away from recommending any of the myriad diets on the market today. *Fat Wars* is not a diet plan; it is designed as a life plan in which you can benefit from your new knowledge on how the body stores and burns fat. However, the confusion in the diet industry concerns not only the calorie allotment of foods, but also the macronutrient profile of these foods. For best results in applying the *Fat Wars* eating principles, I have found that the carbohydrate content, the dietary fat content and the dietary protein content should all be in ratios that are optimal for fat-fighting effect. I have analyzed many of the so-called best macronutrient profiles when it comes to the leading diets, and the one that works the best for the majority of the population seems to be the 40-30-30 plan.

The 40-30-30 plan refers to the breakdown of the various macronutrients in the ratio of carbohydrates (40% of each meal); dietary fat (no more than 30%) and dietary protein (30%). This way of eating was first popularized by Dr. Barry Sears, author of the best-selling *The Zone*, but Dr. Sears was not the one who invented this strategy, which takes into account that eating is indeed a hormonal event. I have mentioned the many disorders in addition to fat gain that the hormone insulin can cause. In order for an eating strategy to be successful for lifelong fat loss, it must take into consideration the effect that foods have on insulin. This is one of the reasons why I do not believe in a high-carbohydrate diet; our prehistoric ancestors (with whom we share 99.99% of our genes) consumed a balance of foods closer to the 40-30-30 way of eating. *Fat Wars* recommends following this eating profile as closely as possible at each meal:

- 40% from carbohydrate sources (minimizing items such as starches and sugars from processed foods, white breads, pasta and polished rice, and maximizing low-glycemic foods such as certain vegetables, legumes, fruits and some whole grains). Carbs provide fuel in the form of glucose (blood sugar) for both brain and muscle activity.

- 30% from dietary fat sources (minimizing items such as butter, cheese, egg yolks, beef fat, lard, trans fats, margarine, french fries and potato chips, and maximizing fats from the omega-3 and omega-6 family such as flaxseed oil, fish oils, olive oil, nuts and avocados). Fats assist in the balance of blood sugar, provide raw materials for hormones, create fuel for long-term energy and strengthen cell walls and mucous membranes.
- 30% from dietary protein sources such as lean meat, chicken breast, fish, low-fat cottage cheese, soy and whey. Dietary proteins help to stabilize blood sugar; promote cell growth and repair; assist hormone production; assist in enzyme production (digestive and metabolic), neurotransmitter production, cell metabolism, body fluid balancing; and maintain the immune system.

In order to keep muscle tissue at optimum levels and assist the body in maintaining all of its other functions, the body must remain in a constant anabolic (growth-promoting) environment. Following these general principles when eating will ensure maximum anabolic effects.

CIRCADIAN EATING RHYTHMS

Circadian rhythms refer to the natural daily patterns of the various processes within our bodies. These are often triggered by the cycle of daylight and darkness. The levels of the human growth hormone rise and fall in a fairly standard rhythmic pattern throughout the day and night, peaking when we're in our deepest phases of sleep. The male hormone testosterone peaks in the morning and then slowly falls. Almost every biochemical function that occurs naturally has a corresponding circadian response. Hunger and eating cycles are no different.

Since we produce most of our energy in the daytime and begin to shut down at night for the sleep phase, eating should follow closely this metabolic cycle. Why would you eat little or nothing for breakfast when you want to produce a great deal of energy in the morning? For that matter, why would you eat an enormous dinner when you are going to be fast asleep not too soon after? This is where many of us lose the battle in the Fat Wars.

In order to take advantage of our natural rhythm of fuelling and activity, we must realize that most of our fat will be burned during the waking hours when our metabolism is at its highest. Therefore, we should eat according to the rate at which our metabolism is able to utilize the fuel sources.

And since metabolism is at its highest in the daytime, with the morning being the best time to start burning fat, then the largest meal should be consumed early in the day instead of at the end.

Here in modern North America we attack this in a backward fashion. Many people think that if they skip breakfast, then they will have one less meal in their system to make them fat. Wrong! This is like starting a long car trip without any fuel in the tank. The body needs fuel in the morning to rev up its engine. (Working out first thing in the morning after the night's fast will rev it up even more. It's the best time to get those fat-burning hormones working for hours afterwards.)

People usually make the mistake of eating not only the wrong *amounts* of food, but also the wrong *kinds* of foods throughout the day. Think of a typical breakfast of sugar-laden cereal or fried goodies, which are all high in high-glycemic carbs and the wrong types of dietary fats. These foods, as we have noted, will shut off your fat-burning machinery for hours, and your fat-burning success is only as good as your last meal. These same people come home from work famished and usually sit down to their biggest meal of the day, which again consists of the wrong foods. Soon afterwards, it's bedtime, usually still on a full tummy, and guess what? Your body now has ample time to store fat until the wee hours of the morning.

So here are some suggestions for eating the *Fat Wars* way:

- The largest meals should be consumed in the morning with the size of these meals declining throughout the day. No one meal should be higher than 500 calories. I have found that it is always best to leave the stomach less full rather than too full. That way, the stomach has an easier time mixing its digestive juices, allowing for a more efficient digestion of the food. The evening meal should be approximately 300–350 calories and should have little or no carbohydrate source other than approved vegetables. This is because high insulin works in opposition to HGH. Eating the right vegetables will allow low-glycemic carbs into the system without disturbing the HGH cycle. The low insulin response to your last meal is the key to burning fat all night long.
- Try to eat every two and a half to three and a half hours for optimum fat burning.
- At least two of the meals should consist of *Fat Wars* Shakes, which contain quality dietary protein, fruit from the berry family (preferably blueberries) or the melon family. Ten shake recipes are included in this chapter, with their macronutrient profiles. (If you work out in the morning, one of the shakes should be consumed immediately after working out.)

- It is very important to stick to foods that are on the low side of the *Fat Wars* Glycemic Index. If you follow this rule with the rest of the *Fat Wars* plan, success can be expected. Since dietary proteins are the key metabolic enhancer of the macronutrients, it's also very important to consume dietary proteins at every meal. In addition, at least 15 mL/1 tbsp of organic flaxseed oil should be consumed per day to supply your body with essential fatty acids to help burn body fat.

FAT WARS SHAKES

Purchasing a powerful blender could be one of the best investments you ever make. By using whole fruits as your base and adding water for the appropriate consistency, you will be adding great-tasting phytonutrition to your diet the way nature intended it to be delivered.

A Word About Juicing

These days everyone seems to be into juicing. We are bombarded by infomercials on how healthy juicing is for us. I'm not here to rain on your parade or anyone else's, for that matter, but the fact is that juicing isn't for everyone. Throughout *Fat Wars*, I have mentioned the myriad of problems associated with high blood sugar levels and their effects on insulin—the hormone with the most impact on our metabolism. This is why I am emphatic about reducing your consumption of high-glycemic or fast-releasing carbohydrates and sticking to more complex ones, such as those found in fresh organic fruits and vegetables.

As I noted in Chapter 6, all carbohydrates eventually break down into sugar in the body. It doesn't matter whether you consume 60 mL/¼ cup of pure sugar or eat a baked potato. They both are 60 mL of sugar to your body, and your body will take the appropriate steps to bring the sugar level back into balance. The body works best with a very small margin of blood sugar, and anything that upsets this balance spells trouble for the entire system.

Your body usually works best with a glucose range of about 90–100 mg/dl (milligrams per deciliter) of blood. When you consume foods like fruit juice, especially without the natural skin and pulp of the fruit, you are supplying pure sugar to your already overworked system. Fruit is not meant to be stripped of its skin and pulp. The skin is usually where most of those important phytochemical flavonoids are found. (Fruit juice will also increase the calorie value of the shakes without providing other valuable nutrients. Remember, we are trying not to go over the 500-calorie mark with each meal, including the *Fat Wars* Shakes.) The only time I would recommend pure juice is with the *Fat Wars* Shake after your workout. This is the one time that your body shouldn't have any problems processing the sugars into stored glycogen instead of stored fat.

Please don't get me wrong. I am not trying to stop you from drinking fruit juice. Instead, I want you to be aware that fruit juice, in enough quantity and like most everything else, can also become fat in your body, thanks to the body's miraculous biochemistry. What I suggest, instead of using pure juice, is to try blended whole fruit.

A Word About "Natural" Sweeteners

Some manufacturers try to gain leverage in the market by using sweeteners that supposedly are as natural as they come, such as fructose, commonly found in fruit sugar. Once again, don't be fooled! Fructose found in fruit is actually good for us; it's when you take it out of its natural environment (fruit) and use it as a sweetener that it begins to cause trouble. In 1998, Dr. Levi and Dr. Werman did a study using rats fed a fructose-rich diet. The results showed that these rats had higher levels of damaged hemoglobin (which interferes with the red blood cells' ability to carry oxygen) and higher levels of lipid peroxidation (which increases oxidation of fatty membranes by free radicals) than in rats fed a sucrose or glucose diet.

Our most prominent connective protein, collagen, can be damaged by cross-linking it through high fructose consumption. Other findings suggest that long-term fructose consumption may actually accelerate the aging cycle. Fructose is hidden in many processed foods and beverages in the form of high-fructose corn syrup. Many nutritionists recommend fructose as an alternative to sucrose for individuals with diabetes or reactive hypoglycemia, since fructose does not cause drastic fluctuations in blood sugar levels. Life is too precious to take chances especially when there are "true" natural alternatives to take advantage of. It's best to support the companies that make the extra effort in trying to bring you, the consumer, the healthiest of ingredients.

By using naturally flavored dietary protein formulas, you will be able to cut down on overall calorie consumption without sacrificing nutrient intake. If you need fruit juice to give your shakes a sweeter taste, try diluting the juice—use half juice and half water—and remember to use your discretion when choosing your beverages. One final note concerning the *Fat Wars* Shakes: remember that nothing takes the place of good, clean water.

Shake Recipes

When adding various ingredients suggested, such as fruit or yogurt, try to use organic products whenever you can. The nutrient content, as well as the lack of contaminants, will be well worth the extra cost. The following is a list of 10 of my most popular protein shakes. All of them are under 500 calories and therefore take advantage of maximum fat-burning potential. They are also balanced to contain all three of the macronutrients for maximum satiety (fullness) potential. Try each of them or come up with your own. Either way, these liquid meals will supply your body with the high-octane fuel it needs to build muscle and burn fat. Enjoy!

Shake Tip #1: When mixing specialized dietary protein isolates, make sure to mix them up first in a shaker cup to avoid harming the delicate protein bonds. Then add them to the shake as the last ingredient and blend only for a few seconds on low speed (just enough to have them mixed in). This will ensure that the high-quality dietary protein will reach your body undenatured.

Shake Tip #2: The macronutrient values listed with each shake give the approximate value of each nutrient. These recipes are not intended to be followed to the letter. Use your own discretion when making these shakes. Based on your individual dietary protein needs, which you will calculate in Chapter 14, you may need to increase or decrease the amounts. I have tried my best to give you a pretty fair guideline to follow, however.

Shake Tip #3: Even though the consistency is liquid, always chew your shake for a few moments before swallowing. This will ensure maximum digestion since digestion starts in the mouth through saliva. After all, food can't help us lose fat if it isn't digested and absorbed effectively.

The base for the *Fat Wars* shakes contains:
- 25–30 g/1 oz (dietary protein content) unflavoured or natural vanilla-flavoured protein isolate powder (whey, soy or mixed)
- 15 mL/1 tbsp flaxseed oil
- 350 mL/1½ cups water

Combine these ingredients in a shaker cup. Shake until smooth.

For:	Blend/Add shake base to:	Approx. Values
FAT WARS BLUES	250 mL/1 cup blueberries 125 mL/½ cup blueberry low-fat yogurt 125 mL/½ cup water	Calories: 445 Protein: 30 g Carbs: 43 g EFAs: 14 g
BLACK AND BLUE	125 mL/½ cup blackberries 125 mL/½ cup blueberries 125 mL/½ cup water	Calories: 450 Protein: 30 g Carbs: 25 g EFAs: 14 g

BOYS ARE BACK IN TOWN	250 mL/1 cup boysenberries 125 mL/½ cup water	Calories: 316 Protein: 25 g Carbs: 25 g EFAs: 14 g
CRANAPPLE SOUR	1 medium apple 250 mL/1 cup cranberries 125 mL/½ cup water	Calories: 378 Protein: 25 g Carbs: 41 g EFAs: 14 g
TANGY TEASE	250 mL/1 cup fresh grapefruit juice 250 mL/1 cup gooseberries	Calories: 480 Protein: 30 g Carbs: 45 g EFAs: 14 g
GREEN BERETS	125 mL/½ cup fresh-squeezed orange juice 1 banana 2 kiwis	Calories: 485 Protein: 30 g Carbs: 68 g EFAs: 14 g
STRAWBERRY BATTLEFIELDS	250 mL/1 cup strawberries 125 mL/½ cup low-fat strawberry yogurt 125 mL/½ cup water	Calories: 415 Protein: 30 g Carbs: 38 g EFAs: 14 g
CRAZY FEELIN'	250 mL/1 cup pineapple 250 mL/1 cup watermelon 125 mL/½ cup water	Calories: 430 Protein: 30 g Carbs: 47 g EFAs: 14 g
MELLOW MELON	250 mL/1 cup fresh-squeezed orange juice 250 mL/1 cup diced cantaloupe	Calories: 435 Protein: 30 g Carbs: 45 g EFAs: 14 g
ENERGY EDGE	125 mL/½ cup fresh-squeezed orange juice 250 mL/1 cup pineapple 250 mL/1 cup blueberries	Calories: 489 Protein: 30 g Carbs: 58 g EFAs: 14 g

For Athletes or Intensive Exercisers

If you are an athlete or a high-intensity exerciser and you are using one of these shakes as a post-workout shake, then eliminate the flaxseed oil and add approximately 50 g/2 oz of a carbohydrate mix. You can find many dry carbohydrate formulas containing glucose polymers on the market. One scoop usually contains approximately 50 g/2 oz of carbohydrate.

12

Top Ten Supplements
For Fat Loss

We hear it all the time: "All you need to do is eat right and you won't need supplements." Nothing could be further from the truth. Low-quality nutrition contributes to disease, low energy levels and obesity. If you think poor nutrition is limited to some Third World country, guess again. Recent research conducted by the U.S. Department of Agriculture shows that the nutrient value of our crops in North America is significantly less than it was just twenty years ago and getting worse by the decade. We've sucked the nutrients out of the soil, and if the plants don't get these nutrients, we don't either. What we need is a second food revolution.

Our failing food system can be revived—if we start to breed crops to extract more nutrients from the soil; increase the diversity of food crops; reduce the loss of nutrients that occur with current harvesting and manufacturing practices; and change the selection of foods we consume to allow for better nutrient absorption. Until then, it's time to get realistic about our diets and admit that often what we eat does more harm than good. My advice—and the advice of many other researchers and professionals in the health field—is to take out cellular insurance by consuming specific supplements that contain one or a variety of special nutrients that aid the body's ability to neutralize toxins and carcinogens, fight free radical damage and help to produce energy and increase metabolism to burn fat. A smart supplement regimen, along with healthy foods, proper exercise and sufficient rest, will go a long way to help you win the Fat Wars.

While there are no magic pills out there, there are a number of effective nutrients that can help to increase our ability to burn fat as long as other lifestyle factors like diet and exercise are taken into consideration. I have carefully researched the top supplements available today pertaining to weight loss, and have listed the top ten supplements that could serve as your allies in the Fat Wars.

Supplements are reinforcements that help guarantee victory. While each fat-burning nutrient or combination of nutrients listed helps to improve (directly or indirectly) the function of muscle cells, fat-burning lipolytic enzymes, transport proteins and mitochondrion, some can do a lot more than fight fat. The goal is to prevent your muscle cells from becoming sluggish and weak—weighed down with saturated and trans fats, low in fat-burning enzymes and transport proteins and unreceptive to insulin. By taking the various fat-burning nutrients recommended, you'll immediately turn the tide of your personal Fat War in your favor. Specific product recommendations are listed in Appendix II; what follows is a general discussion of the nutrients and what they can do.

Does this mean that you can slack off on your diet, not exercise, get little sleep and still lose lots of fat? NO! Remember: there are no magic pills, just the right combinations of all the necessary lifestyle factors to guarantee a victory.

For People with Diabetes

Some of the nutrients listed can improve the sensitivity of muscle cells to insulin. By making the cells more receptive to insulin, less insulin is needed. Less insulin means more fat-burning enzymes, transport proteins and healthy mitochondrion. And if you are an over-fat person with Type 2 diabetes, you'll find these nutrients very helpful in controlling your blood sugar level, reducing your percentage of damaged, oxygen-carrying hemoglobin, and melting the fat. What a bonus! However, a word of caution is in order. These cell-sensitizing agents can have a profound influence on lowering blood sugar levels. If you are on blood sugar-lowering medications such as insulin, Metformin and/or sulfonylureas, using some of the nutrients listed may require you to reduce your medications in order to avoid hypoglycemia (low blood sugar). I have seen this more often than not. If you have concerns, or if you have diabetes, consult your physician or diabetes educator before using these nutrients.

PROTEIN ISOLATES

The key to long-term fat loss is building healthy muscle cells that can accept the fat and burn it up. All of the key structures to accomplish fat burning are protein based, so it's critical to ingest enough protein at regular intervals during the day. Nothing accomplishes this task better than high-quality protein. Fortunately, we can incorporate high-quality proteins into our diet quickly and easily. Dietary protein powder isolates can be mixed with just about anything to create a high-powered protein shake in minutes.

These protein isolates enable our bodies to rebuild and repair themselves (anabolism) faster than ever before. Anabolism creates the optimum environment for proper muscle recovery not only from workouts, but also from the everyday stresses of life. The more effective your body becomes at anabolism, the better equipped your body will be to burn off unwanted fat.

The two top protein isolates available today are high-alpha whey and non-GMO soy.

Whey Protein Isolates

Whey protein, the formerly useless by-product of cheese production, has now become the highest quality protein known to science. It is a high-quality protein that can be fat- and lactose-free. Here are some of the many advantages of whey protein isolates over other protein sources:

- It exits the stomach faster than other protein sources, providing a substantial and rapid rise in blood amino acids for enhanced anabolism.
- Lactose-free forms of whey enable those with lactose intolerance to benefit from whey's superior amino acid profile.
- It helps to stimulate the release of the hormone glucagon, which stimulates fat burning.
- It stimulates the liver's release of special polypeptides called somatomedins or insulin-like growth factors, which control the rate of muscle growth.
- In clinical settings, whey has been shown to increase the immune response by up to 500% due to its high levels of the amino acid L-cysteine.
- Whey contains a small protein compound called glycomacropeptide (GMP), which decreases appetite levels by stimulating the release of an appetite-suppressing hormone (cholecystokinin or CCK). In recent studies, GMPs from whey protein were shown to raise CCK by a whopping 415%.

There are a number of different types of whey protein on the market, and it is important that you become a smart consumer. Quality whey isolates are extremely expensive to produce so many companies blend their formulas with cheaper concentrates. If you're buying whey protein and want the GMPs, remember that the cross-flow membrane-extracted whey is the only version that contains them.

It is also important to look for a high fraction of whey called alpha-lactalbumin. The alpha portion of whey constitutes the major component of mother's milk (up to 25%), hence its amazing anabolic activity. This low molecular weight fraction is quickly absorbed into the system, allowing for better repair of the muscle tissue. High-alpha whey isolates have also been shown to increase one of our most important antioxidants—glutathione—more effectively than anything else. The higher the glutathione levels in the body, the healthier we are.

Soy Protein Isolates

Soy proteins were the first protein powders available as a supplement. However, previous extraction technology did not allow soy to be isolated effectively, which destroyed most of the beneficial isoflavones (plant hormones) in soy. Newer isolation methods allow for an incredible protein isolate that retains an abundance of these tiny, powerful, heart-disease fighters, cancer fighters and fat-loss helpers.

Soy isolates also contain some of nature's highest quantities of branched-chain amino acids (BCAAs) and glutamine. BCAAs and glutamine make up the majority of amino acids in muscle tissue and provide fuel for muscle function and repair. Here are some of the many advantages of soy protein isolates over other protein sources:

- It can increase metabolic activity by increasing thyroid hormone production.
- It has been shown to be effective in lowering the insulin-to-glucagon ratio.
- It contains the special phytochemicals/isoflavones genestein and diadzein, which have a variety of potent effects on the body, including inhibiting certain types of cancer.
- It has been shown to increase bone density in postmenopausal women by increasing estrogen levels and reducing the formation of osteoclasts (the cells that degrade bone).
- It can inhibit cardiovascular disease by reducing platelet aggregation and the oxidation of low-density lipoproteins (LDLs).
- It can also act as a natural diuretic because the isoflavones increase kidney function.
- It can help menopausal women lose fat by acting as estrogen supporters (see Chapter 4, "Her Fat").

The quality of the soy protein you choose can make all the difference—the key is its active isoflavone content. Most soy proteins are poorly produced; manufacturers use alcohol extraction, which removes most (if not all) of the active isoflavones. Many mass-produced soy products, including tofu, also lose vast amounts of their isoflavones during processing.

The traditional Japanese process of fermenting soy foods retains their isoflavone content and even enhances the activity of the isoflavones. When it comes to soy protein powders, only water-extracted soy protein isolate will retain its natural isoflavone advantage. It is also very important to choose a non-GMO soy isolate, since according to the U.S. Department of Agriculture, over 57% of soy products currently on the market are from genetically modified soy. If the packaging doesn't list this important feature, it is likely from a genetically altered source. Please read your labels!

Other Benefits of Protein Isolates

Both whey and soy have unique qualities to assist you in attaining the physique you've always wanted. You can take either one of these proteins alone, or combine them for maximum benefit (a combined version of the two is listed in Appendix II). One of the benefits of consuming high-quality whey, soy or a mix of the two isolates is that you are guaranteed the exact amount of protein you need, without the added fat and carbohydrates—a definite bonus for any fat-loss program. This is the best way to fine-tune your dieting strategy. Together, the right kind of soy and whey isolates can offer an effective insurance policy against the breakdown (catabolic processes) of the body.

ESSENTIAL FATTY ACIDS (EFAS)

As we discussed in Chapter 7, when it comes to the optimum functioning of your fat-burning machinery, it takes fat to burn fat. Feeding the body the wrong types of fats makes the cells dysfunctional (and lousy fat burners). We need to supply our bodies with friendly fat allies that we cannot make on our own—the right amount of these essential fats keeps the cells happy and helps them burn more fat. Those essential fats are omega-6 and omega-3, which are found in an optimum regular diet or taken in supplement form.

Omega-6 (linoleic acid) can be found in polyunsaturated safflower, sunflower, cottonseed and corn oils, and is also present in high amounts in foods such as walnuts, wheat germ and soybeans. Of approximately 50 essential nutrients, omega-6 has the highest daily requirement—around 3–6% of calories (15 mL/1 tbsp) per day. Omega-6 plus an enzyme transforms into gamma-linolenic acid (GLA), another helpful dietary fat found in the oils of evening primrose, borage and black currant seeds. Research seems to support the addition of either evening primrose or borage oils for their preformed gamma linolenic acid (GLA) content ensures that our bodies have enough of this important fatty acid. As discussed in Chapter 7, arachidonic acid (AA), a cousin of omega-6, is in meats, eggs and dairy products, but too much AA can cause increased inflammation in the body. Therefore, if you have some form of arthritis, it is best to cut down on these AA-containing foods.

Omega-3 (alpha-linolenic acid) can be found in large amounts in flaxseed oil and meal, and in lesser amounts in canola oil and hemp seed oil. Omega-3, like omega-6, has the ability to be transformed into closely related friendly fats such as eicosapentaenoic acid (EPA) and docosahexaenoic acid (DHA). Research has shown that omega-3 fatty acids help to improve brain function. (DHA is an essential fatty acid for the growth and functional development of the brain in infants.) Omega-3 fats are also able to help us lose body fat. One of the omega-3 fatty acids (EPA) lowers blood levels of triglycerides by increasing the transport of fatty acids into the cells for fat burning (thermogenesis).

Large quantities of omega-3 fats can also be found preformed in wild, cold-water fish such as Atlantic cod, Pacific halibut, sole, menhaden, mackerel, rockfish, salmon and tuna. (Farm-raised fish such as salmon do not contain enough of these preformed omega-3s, likely because their diet is devoid of omega-3s.)

Marine oils are very reactive and must be protected from heat, sunlight and oxygen. EFAs are required in gram amounts daily and are highly perishable, deteriorating rapidly when exposed to air, light, heat and metals.

If you choose to supplement your diet with extra EFAs, I recommend that you take 1 tbsp/15 mL of cold-pressed organic flaxseed oil and 1 tsp/ 5 mL of cold-pressed organic borage oil with your *Fat Wars* Shake every day. In addition, take 1 capsule of molecularly distilled (i.e., no PCBs or mercury toxicity) cold-water (Norwegian or North Atlantic) fish oil with each meal.

CONCENTRATED GREEN FOODS

Nutrition researchers have always told us to eat our fruits and vegetables. Fruits and vegetables contain the phytonutrients (plant chemicals) that are capable of exerting powerful, positive effects on our bodies. Even the simple soybean, tomato or blueberry is a miracle of complexity. We presently estimate that there are 30,000–50,000 bioenergetic phytonutrients in plants; only 1,000 of these have been isolated so far, and only about 100 of these disease-preventing plant compounds have been analyzed and tested.

When you use plants as your food and energy source, you eat foods that are alive with energy. If you use animals as your food source, then you obtain the energy of plants indirectly, since the plant nutrients are converted by the animals; the animal nutrients are then converted into the tissues, cells, atoms and subatomic particles of your body. Life energy from bioenergetic whole foods not only gives you energy, but also keeps you in healthful balance (anabolic capacity) by preventing either the initiation or promotion of degenerative diseases.

Whole plant-based foods are grown in sunlight and infused with the energy of the soil and water; they can increase your energy, improve moods and motivation and help to decrease your appetite. They can boost your metabolic rate and help to increase your body's fat-burning machinery by reviving your energetic, anabolic drive.

It is recommended that we consume six to 10 servings of organic fruits and vegetables every day to obtain the maximum benefits from these plants. The reality, however, is that very few of us actually do this. This is why concentrated green food powders are highly recommended in the *Fat Wars* Plan. And with green food concentrates, all you have to do is drink them.

Look for only the highest-quality green food concentrates that contain a mixture of organic land and sea vegetables, as well as a mixture of synergistic herbs. The powder can be mixed quite easily in a shaker cup (usually provided), and should be consumed either between meals or with a protein shake; some actually come premixed with protein isolates (see Appendix II).

ANTIOXIDANTS

Antioxidants play a role in burning your body fat. Without them, your chances of dropping the fat are greatly reduced.

While oxygen is necessary for life, it can also harm cells. Antioxidants are produced by the body and are also present in many foods. They enable our cells to function properly by protecting them from free radicals: unstable molecules that can damage cell structures and lead to cell death. Cell processes such as energy production, as well as exposure to smoke, pollutants, solar radiation and even aerobic exercise, constantly produce free radicals. Ninety-five percent of the free radical production takes place in the muscle's energy center, the mitochondrion (where fat is burned), so it is very important to protect these energy centers from undue damage.

Scientists have identified 1,100 varieties of these free radicals to date. Recent research confirms that various antioxidants work together, each supporting the other, in stopping cell-damaging free radicals in their tracks. Just as free radicals work in combinations, attacking us from every which way, antioxidants must also work in synergy with one another to stop the onslaught.

Although there are probably hundreds of antioxidants, research has shown that the most effective (as a family) are vitamins C and E, lipoic acid (thiotic acid), glutathione (GSH) and Coenzyme Q10 (CoQ10). Dr. Lester Packer and his researchers at the University of California at Berkeley call them network antioxidants. The network antioxidants work together as a team. The right combination of these antioxidants and others not a part of the core team will contribute to your total cell health and maximum fat-burning ability.

Vitamin C: Vitamin C is a potent water-soluble vitamin that protects the watery interior of the cells. Since it belongs to the water-soluble family of nutrients, any excess is excreted in the urine. The only negative effects of too high a consumption of vitamin C are diarrhea and cramping, which is often temporary and certainly not a great health risk.

The researcher who placed vitamin C at the forefront of antioxidants was the late Dr. Linus Pauling, whose work is being supported today by new research showing the beneficial effects of this antioxidant team player. Studies of vitamin C suggest that it can help prevent cancer, lower the risk of cardiovascular disease and improve collagen production. In addition, over-fat and obese individuals, as well as people with Type 2 diabetes, require more vitamin C because they excrete it more quickly. It does not take a lot of vitamin C to get the job done. Recent research shows that a dose of about 200 mg results in half of it being excreted, unchanged, in the urine. If the dose is 2 g, the amount excreted rises to 90%. Because the body seems to reach a certain saturation point, it makes sense to take a smaller dose of vitamin C more often. I suggest that you take 200–500 mg at a time, two or three times daily.

Although they are not part of the antioxidant family, I also recommend a good quality, full spectrum B complex supplement each day because the B vitamins are involved in the metabolism of proteins, carbohydrates and fats, as well as a high-quality, multimineral complex for added benefit.

How to Take Your Antioxidants

Antioxidants are nutrients (as are vitamins and minerals) and most nutrients are best absorbed with food. Always take your antioxidants with the appropriate foods. If the nutrients are fat-soluble like vitamin E, CoQ10 or the carotenoid family (beta carotene, lycopene, etc.), then they should be taken with food containing fats such as the omega-6s and omega-3s. All the antioxidants can be taken together.

Vitamin E: Vitamin E is a terrific antiaging antioxidant that improves the immune system, protects against sun damage, relieves arthritic symptoms and makes strong cell walls. Vitamin E is a fat-soluble antioxidant, which means it can go places where water-soluble antioxidants can't. As it is fat-soluble, you can acquire high concentrations of this vitamin because it stays in the body much longer than water-soluble vitamins do. Excess amounts of vitamin E (over 1600 iu) can be toxic. Two of the most important functions of vitamin E involve its action on fat-soluble structures—the cell wall itself and the blood- and cell-based fatty acids, which include LDL cholesterol and triglycerides (fats).

Vitamin E breaks the chain of free radicals acting on lipids, preventing the spread of free radicals that can damage lipids and proteins. Research shows that it takes a minimum of 400 iu of vitamin E daily to protect LDL cholesterol from oxidation. In addition, vitamin E is shown to stop free radical reactions from increasing the risk of cancers, heart disease, vision problems and oxidative stress due to exercise. Since we are talking about burning excess body fat, we must protect ourselves from excess lipid peroxidation (fats becoming oxidized); nothing will protect against this process better than vitamin E. Vitamin E also works in close relationship with our next antioxidant, lipoic acid.

If you are under the age of 40, take one or two 400 iu capsules a day of oil-based (mixed tocopherol) vitamin E with food that contains some fat. If you are over 40, take one or two 400 iu capsules of dry-based (mixed tocopherol) vitamin E with food that contains some fat.

Lipoic Acid: Lipoic acid is one of the most amazing antioxidants ever discovered. It offers great protection against heart disease, stroke, memory loss and cataracts. It also helps to control blood sugar levels, reducing harmful blood protein-sugar complexes known as advanced glycation end products (AGEs). It's the AGEs that really put the age on people with diabetes because they tend to make large amounts of this substance. So what's the problem with AGEs? They create free radicals that wreak havoc on cells, nerves and connective tissue. This is a big reason why people with diabetes are at a high risk for kidney failure, blindness and/or poor circulation.

Lipoic acid also protects our genetic structures—DNA from damage and mutation, and the intracellular mitochondrion from damage. Remember: the mitochondrion in your muscle cells are the powerhouse of fat burning. If your mitochondrion becomes overly damaged by increased free radical damage, you can kiss your permanent fat-burning plan goodbye. Lipoic acid is a team player. It's both fat soluble and water soluble, so it can go anywhere. It can also recycle other antioxidants like vitamins C and E CoQ10, and even itself.

Lipoic acid is critical for optimal energy production because it helps convert sugar (glucose) into usable energy for ATP resynthesis, enabling your fat-burning cells to fire up the furnaces. When lipoic acid stops a free radical in its tracks, the lipoic acid itself becomes a weak free radical, but don't worry—it regenerates itself into action again. It's the only antioxidant known to do this. You should consume 100 mg or more of lipoic acid per day. According to the latest research, lipoic acid should be taken throughout the day because it doesn't last all day in our systems. It is recommended to start with 50 mg twice daily. If you are really exercising hard, smoke (I hope you'll quit and replace it with exercise) or are exposed to a greater number of pollutants (i.e., the big city), you should increase your consumption of lipoic acid to 100–150 mg twice daily. Your fat-burning muscle cells and their internal army of anti-fat warriors will love you for it. Take 50–100 mg of lipoic acid (also known as alpha-lipoic acid) two or three times a day, approximately half an hour away from food for best results.

Glutathione

Glutathione is well documented as the most important and abundant antioxidant that is naturally produced by the body. Even so, the body still needs glutathione's precursors to build enough of it. Throughout the bloodstream and the cells, glutathione neutralizes free radicals and removes toxins. Not only does glutathione boost the immune system, but research has shown that it has an essential role in improving liver function, preventing cancer, promoting longevity, alleviating bronchitis and psoriasis, producing energy and generally preventing disease.

Glutathione is a tripeptide (a peptide is a small protein) made of three amino acids. Of the three amino acids—cysteine, glycine and glutamic acid—cysteine is the most important since it contains the crucial sulfur molecule needed to form glutathione. It is not necessary to take pure glutathione in pill form since it has been shown to break down through digestion, but it is nonetheless important. The best natural way to boost glutathione levels in the body is by ingesting lipoic acid and high-alpha whey protein isolates (see Appendix II for AlphaPure™). High-alpha whey proteins can contain up to 2.5 times the cysteine levels present in other whey protein isolates, which makes them an excellent and unsurpassed source of natural glutathione builders.

Coenzyme Q10: An enzyme is a protein that brings about specific chemical reactions; a coenzyme works with the enzyme to produce a reaction. CoQ10 is a coenzyme that helps to produce the energy that keeps cells functioning properly. It's found in high amounts in the mitochondrion, where it helps to make ATP and acts as a protective, fat-soluble antioxidant.

Along with vitamin E, CoQ10 plays a free radical defense role by riding along with lipoproteins in the bloodstream, protecting fatty acids from attack by free radicals. Because energy is so very important in the proper functioning of your muscle cells, especially when it comes to disease prevention and burning fat, you'll want to take some supplemental CoQ10 to keep your mitochondrion protected and your cells humming along nicely. Remember: a healthy, active cell is a fat-burning cell.

CoQ10 is available as a powder or a gel. The gel is reported to be better absorbed and raises the blood levels of CoQ10. Because CoQ10 can be expensive, a small dose should do the trick without emptying your wallet. Take 30–60 mg a day of oil-based CoQ10 with foods that contain some fat.

For best results and convenience in general, look for antioxidant preparations that include the whole family of network antioxidants (see Appendix II).

Support Antioxidants
I've addressed various key antioxidants, but there are others that are still of great value to your antioxidant arsenal. These include selenium, zinc, manganese and plant-based compounds called flavonoids. The flavonoids are of particular value as they can boost the effectiveness of vitamin C, glutathione and the other antioxidants mentioned earlier. Flavonoids are also shown to improve the health of blood vessels, promote good circulation and the transport of important nutrients, treat impotence, strengthen the immune system, reduce inflammation and boost memory and learning.

Flavonoids: Berries such as bilberry, blueberry and blackberry all contain valuable flavonoids, as does the spice turmeric, which has a potent antioxidant known as curcumin. There are hundreds of different flavonoids in plants; some have been well researched and commercial nutrients have been developed. Concentrated sources of flavonoids include ginko biloba, grape seed, bilberry, hawthorne berry, curcumin and pine bark extracts, all of which are generally available through health food stores and drug stores. Some plant extracts are more expensive than others.

- Ginko biloba is most noted for its powerful memory-boosting abilities, but it also has much value as a cortisol reducer. In a recent study, ginko biloba inhibited cortisol production very effectively.

Remember: less cortisol equals more muscle and less fat. A good dose would be at least 30 mg taken twice a day.

- Quality full-spectrum grape extract formulas should contain 95% procyanidolic values with resveratrol and ellagic acid. A useful dosage would be 60 mg, taken two or three times a day with meals.

- Milk thistle, with its key ingredient silymarin, is one of the most effective nutrients for regenerating liver function. What would the liver possibly have to do with burning body fat? The liver is the main metabolic organ in the body, and liver cells are responsible for carbohydrate, fat and protein metabolism. A healthy and happy liver cell can become an especially efficient fat burner, firing up the furnaces to churn through excess fatty acids. The flavonoids in milk thistle also protect the liver cells from free radical damage (it's a potent antioxidant). As well, flavonoids have anti-cancer effects, improve insulin sensitivity (it lowers insulin levels) and reduce excess cortisol levels. Generally, standardized milk thistle extracts contain a minimum of 75% silymarin. At this potency, a dose of 50–100 mg two or three times daily will really boost liver cell activity and keep your fat-burning army marching along toward victory.

CHROMIUM

As we've already discussed, high blood sugar levels result in a spike in the hormone insulin, leading to cellular disruption and obesity. More than 90% of North Americans are deficient in chromium. When you combine low chromium consumption with high blood sugar levels due to a high consumption of sweets, breads and refined foods, the result is a staggering increase in Type 2 diabetes, over-fatness and obesity. Most soils contain little or no chromium. As a result, the plants we eat contain very little chromium. The best way to boost the level of chromium in your cells is to take a supplement.

If you are over-fat, there is a good chance you are insulin resistant. Your cells just don't let the sugar enter their interiors as well as they used to. This results in the pro-fat insulin spike that keeps the fat pounds on despite vigorous exercise and diet routines. Chromium is essential to reducing the cells' resistance to insulin. It helps your cells function better, allowing blood sugar and amino acids in and keeping blood insulin levels lower.

Chromium is usually a very hard mineral to absorb effectively, but two of the most popular forms of chromium, chromium polynicotinate (niacin-bound chromium) and chromium picolinate, should both perform well and have been researched extensively. A recent study comparing the two forms of chromium in conjunction with exercise gave the nod to niacin-bound chromium. The recommended dosage is 200–400 mcg (micrograms) of elemental chromium per day.

CITRUS AURANTIUM

Citrus aurantium is a natural stimulant that is derived from the essential oils of the bitter Seville orange. This herb has been used for thousands of years to improve circulation and liver function and treat indigestion.

Increased resting metabolic rate means more fat calories burned. The fat-burning effect results from a group of compounds in the herb called adrenergic amines (organic compounds that are able to release or behave like adrenaline or noradrenaline), with the most effective one for fat-loss being synephrine. Most extracts sold today are standardized for 4% or 6% synephrine. In addition to the flavonoids found in *Citrus aurantium*, this herb has the ability to produce an energizing and fat-burning effect on the body by activating a specific group of cell receptors known as beta-3 receptors. These receptors increase the rate at which fat is released from both fat and muscle cells (lipolysis), and increase the resting metabolic rate (thermogenesis). (You may even feel this herbal extract working as your body will be generating heat.)

Citrus aurantium, unlike the popular fat-burning stimulant ephedra, does not raise pulse rate or blood pressure. The recommended dose of a standardized *Citrus aurantium* 6% synephrine extract is 325 mg per day, taken in divided doses about a half hour before each meal or shake.

HYDROXYCITRIC ACID

A fruit from India called *Garcinia cambogia* contains an important fat-burning chemical called hydroxycitric acid or HCA for short. While research has shown that HCA prevents the conversion of carbohydrates into fat, a more important function of this incredible nutrient is its ability to help increase the special fat-releasing enzyme called carnitine palmitoyl transferase (CPT). The enzyme that converts excess glucose into fat is called ATP-citrate lyase. HCA inhibits this enzyme from making more fat and in the process slows down another enzyme called malonyl-CoA, causing an increase in the levels of CPT (the fat-releasing enzyme).

Another advantage of HCA is that it inhibits glucose-stimulated insulin secretion, which helps to keep this fat-storing hormone in check. HCA has been on the market for a few years now, but the results have been mixed. In the past, the HCA was bound to a calcium salt, which may not have been the best absorbed. Recently a new HCA salt with magnesium (Mg) has come on the market. By adding Mg-HCA to your supplement program, you'll greatly increase the amount of CPT, which will allow for an increase in fat-burning potential. I suggest a dose of 500 mg to 2 g of Mg-HCA (Citrimax) derived from *Garcinia cambogia*, taken in divided doses twice daily, as a very important addition to your fat-burning army.

FORSKOLIN

Forskolin, from the herb *Coleus forskohlii*, increases the levels of the cellular messenger cyclic Adenosine Monophosphate (cAMP), which is a major regulator of fat-burning enzymes and a messenger that reacts with certain hormones to direct certain metabolic changes inside cells. It is a must for anyone interested in boosting the fat-burning rate. Once cAMP is formed inside cells, it stimulates other enzymes that activate additional enzymes (the domino effect). As such, a little cAMP goes a long way; it is increased by high glucagon levels and reduced by high insulin levels. It also stimulates the thyroid hormones catecholamines and glucagon to perform their fat-burning jobs and other metabolic processes.

The release of fatty acids from fat cells is controlled by the activity of the enzyme known as hormone-sensitive lipase (HSL), which is dependent on the intracellular cAMP levels. CAMP is also increased by catecholamines such as adrenaline and noradrenaline. Take a divided dose of 100 mg of *Coleus forskohlii* standardized to contain 10% forskolin (10 mg of forskolin) twice a day.

GREEN TEA EXTRACT

Green tea is beneficial for the mind and body, and can speed up fat loss. Tea is rich in flavonoids called catechins, which are very well absorbed compared with other flavonoids. The catechins are powerful antioxidants and have been shown to inhibit certain cancers, improve blood flow in the cardiovascular system and reduce LDL cholesterol oxidation.

In addition, recent research has shown the catechins in green tea to be thermogenic. Thus green tea extract may also help dieters shed fat, according to research in the December 1999 issue of the *American Journal of Clinical Nutrition*. This is the first human study to examine the influence of tea on energy expenditure and body composition. Green tea may be particularly useful for heart disease patients who are trying to lose weight because, unlike weight-loss drugs, it does not affect the heart rate. Catechin polyphenol compounds work with other chemicals to increase levels of fat oxidation and thermogenesis, helping the body burn fuel such as fat.

If the fat-burning effect of green tea doesn't excite you, here are some other benefits: green tea can lower serum glucose levels by inhibiting the activity of the starch-digesting enzyme amylase, so that starch is absorbed more slowly (insulin levels would also be decreased); green tea has been shown to lower intestinal fat absorption as well. Diphenylamine, another compound in green tea, seems to have a strong sugar-lowering action as well. New research shows that green tea catechins produce one of the strongest vasodilating responses, thus allowing for increased blood flow. An increase in peripheral circulation is valuable for increased oxygenation and therefore increased energy production. If all this wasn't enough, green tea also has the ability to raise brain levels of serotonin and/or dopamine, which control both the appetite and satiety response. Why not just drink green tea? Because standardized extracts of green tea have more of the active compounds than brewed tea alone can offer. I recommend taking 300–400 mg of green tea extract daily, standardized for 50% or more catechins, with a majority being one particular catechin called EGCG.

CARNITINE

Certain nutrients stimulate the actual fat-burning activity inside cells by activating the important enzymes required for the lipolytic process. Carnitine is part of the amino acid family, but works very much like a vitamin. It cannot, however, be classified as a vitamin since it is manufactured in the human body from two amino acids, lysine and methionine. It is also part of the fatty acid transport enzyme carnitine palmitoyl transferase (CPT), which is needed to mobilize fat reserves for energy production (a very good thing). L-carnitine is a natural substance essential for the mitochondrial oxidation of fatty acids; it regulates the energy metabolism of cells. Carnitine is a cofactor that helps transform long-chain fatty acids and then transports them into the mitochondrion where they are burned as fuel. Conditions that seem to benefit from supplemental L-carnitine include anorexia, chronic fatigue, cardiovascular disease, diabetes, male infertility, muscular myopathies and obesity. L-carnitine also regulates the level of Coenzyme A (CoA) in mitochondrion to ensure that energy metabolism is functioning at an optimal rate.

Carnitine is slowly absorbed from the intestines into the bloodstream, and the percentage absorbed is related to the amount ingested. Studies show that out of a 2 g oral dose, only 16% is absorbed and that higher doses do not increase the amount absorbed at one time. This tells us that the body can use just so much L-carnitine at one time. Ingesting carnitine at a dose of 1.5 g twice daily can raise free carnitine by 20% and acetyl-L-carnitine by 80%. Carnitine is concentrated in human breast milk and colostrum (pre-milk breast fluid). Supplementing with bovine colostrum may be a great way to increase carnitine levels.

It is well accepted that high blood sugar levels suppress the burning of fatty acids as energy. While most over-fat and obese persons are doing a good job of freeing up the fatty acids for fuel, those fatty acids just can't get into the mitochondrion to be burned. As a result, they stay around, only to be reformed into triglycerides or stored again in body fat.

The trick to long-term permanent fat loss is to increase the amount and activity of CPT. Proper exercise can double CPT activity, making it a super-efficient catalyst in the fat-burning process. That is another great reason to train regularly. It is also important to reduce insulin and raise glucagon levels by limiting high-glycemic carbohydrates and increasing quality protein consumption. If you decide to add this nutrient to your Fat Wars team, you will need to take at least 500 mg of acetyl-L-carnitine or 1 g of L-carnitine twice a day on an empty stomach for best results.

All of the supplements mentioned will assist you in your victory over body fat, but it's the basic changes in your food intake and activity levels that are key. Whether you choose to take supplements or not—and I do recommend them—it's the combination of changes you make that matter.

13

Getting Physical

As I've mentioned, our bodies developed thousands of years ago. Back then, we walked, ran and climbed to get where we were going and to secure what we needed. We fought for food alongside the many animals that shared our home. Today it's a different story. We take our car to work, sit at a desk for hours and then slump in front of the television for a few hours each night. Boy, is life tough! It may well be mentally tough, but physically tough is another thing. Today we actually have to go out of our way to get physical.

Our metabolism is designed to prepare for those times when we will be on the move. Our bodies save the fuel (fat) for a rainy day—a day that never seems to come any more. In fact, fewer than 30% of North Americans take part in much physical activity, and 25% do none at all, so we get fatter and fatter. Without proper fat-burning exercise, we will never win the Fat Wars.

While all of us value health and physical fitness, many of us have not learned to integrate physical activity into our daily lives. We all know people who exercise consistently, sometimes more than five times a week, week after week. They seem to be different from us. Instead of regarding exercise as a chore, they make it fun and invigorating. For the rest of us, it's another matter. Most of us are great starters. We forge ahead at the beginning of the year, filling up the health clubs on Monday evenings to overflow capacity. But by April, it's business as usual. That health club membership is wasted, that piece of home exercise equipment gathers dust in the corner of the room, that aerobics videotape is buried between *When Harry Met Sally* and *The Terminator*.

If we're going to lose as much fat as possible and keep it off, we have to get moving in the right way. However, the majority of exercise routines developed for weight loss over the past 20 years are not designed to melt away the fat and keep it off.

THE AEROBICS MYTH

Carmen had just turned 30, and with the births of three kids behind her, she felt ready to tackle her next task—dropping the fat that had slowly collected around her waist, hips, butt and thighs over the past decade.

Exercise was nothing new to Carmen. She had already tried a variety of routines at the local community center. She had even ordered a few so-called "miracle" devices from the infomercial channel that seemed too good to be true. They were. Carmen tried walking, but the pounds just didn't seem to budge. She even invested in an abdominal-crunch machine and an aerobics video so she could train at home. After three months of sweating to hip-hop, she felt more energetic, but the fat was still entrenched. What was she doing wrong, and why isn't she alone?

By far, the most common form of physical activity recommended for weight loss is aerobics. We've seen them: those spandex-clad cuties moving and shaking to the music, inviting us to get out on the dance floor and boogie with them. We've also seen the testimonials from those who have succeeded by adding aerobics to their weight-loss program. But the fact is that for every person who has won the war against fat by using aerobics, there are 50 others who have not. The success rate when it comes to permanent fat loss via pure aerobics is not very high.

Many of us have tried aerobics ourselves. Most of us have taken long brisk walks, spent 30–45 minutes on a treadmill or stationary bike, danced to the music of an aerobics class or home video and maybe even tried a Tae-Bo™ class or two. The truth is, aerobic workouts are long, and the fat burned during the workout is minimal. As in dieting and fasting, the engines that actually burn the fat—muscle tissue—is burned up too, and the increase in the amount of fat burned before the next workout is almost zip. Hard-core aerobics is anti-muscle—athletes such as elite 10,000-meter runners or marathon participants carry very little muscle mass. Of course, aerobics proponents have recognized this, and many aerobic classes at gyms and health clubs these days also do some sort of resistance training such as step (using body weight as resistance), or using small hand weights or elastic cords. But these attempts at making up for the deficiencies of aerobic exercise are weak at best. Aerobics are just not the most efficient fat-burning exercises.

BUILD MUSCLE, BURN FAT

In contrast to aerobics, resistance training builds muscle, and it's muscle that is going to help us win the war on fat. Not only do we want to build muscles, we want to turn on the muscles that we already have. Turn them on? Yes, the muscles we already have can actually be tuned up to become more efficient at burning fat. The right type of exercise can do that for us. We'll transform our muscles into the fat-burning army that they are capable of becoming. As the army ads say, "Be all that you can be." In this case, our muscles will burn all that they can burn.

Why are muscles so important? As I have stated throughout, muscles constitute the metabolic engine of the body. The more muscle we carry on our frames, the higher our basal metabolic rate; the more active those muscles are, the more fat we burn, 24 hours each day.

That fat we are packing around is deadweight. Fat is an inert substance—it just sits there taking up space (and it doesn't look that good either). Now here's the most important point—one pound of active muscle burns more than 50 calories a day. So, if we add muscle during our fat loss program, or at least keep the muscle we have, we will be well on our way to winning the Fat Wars. And too much cardio can quickly turn into a muscle-wasting activity.

In a landmark study published in the prestigious *American Journal of Cardiology*, aerobic training was compared to aerobic-with-resistance (weight) training. Participants were split into two groups and had to complete a ten-week exercise program of 75 minutes. One group completed 75 minutes of aerobic exercise twice a week, while the other completed 40 minutes of aerobics plus 35 minutes of weight training. At the end of the study, the aerobics group had an 11% increase in endurance, but no increase in their strength. The group that completed the combination of aerobics-with-resistance training showed a massive 109% increase in their endurance, and a 21–43% increase in their overall strength. There are many other studies that further prove the theory that resistant training with low-impact cardio is superior to either one alone.

The usual scenario is as follows: you have been performing high-intensity cardio for weeks now, but you're no closer to reaching your fat-loss goals. In fact, you seem to have gained an extra pound in the last week. It's time to increase the cardio for better fat-burning effect. Bad move! The more cardio you do, the more likely your body will burn sugar and protein instead of fat. In order to create extra sugar, the body will begin to break down body proteins from muscle in a process called gluconeogenesis (the remaking of sugar from other body materials). Muscle will be lost, fat-burning capacity diminished and the saga continues. This process cannibalizes muscle tissue almost faster than dieting does.

How Hard Do We Have to Work to Burn Fat?

In order to better understand how to train effectively for proper, long-term fat-burning success, we first have to understand what type of fuel source the body is using to do a specific activity. The problem is that most exercise will primarily burn sugar and protein as fuel sources and leave fat alone. Sugars as well as proteins are broken down to their simplest forms for energy more easily than fat is. Fats are made up of many single units called fatty acids. These individual fatty acids must first be broken apart in order to contribute their energy value, a lengthy process—and, as we saw in the discussion of metabolism, many forms of exercise don't get us to fourth gear (the fat-burning one). Most exercise programs touted by the so-called exercise gurus of our generation will tell people to train at 70% of their maximum heart rate for fat loss. The maximum heart rate is measured using that familiar mathematical equation of subtracting our age from the number 220. Training heart rate is calculated by multiplying maximum heart rate by the percentage we want to train at, in this case 70%.

> *Example:* Carmen is 33 years old, so she would calculate her training heart rate as:
> $220 - 33 \times 70\%$ = a training heart rate of 131

The idea behind this training heart rate theory of 70% is that it will allow us to perform the most effective level of exercise—the one where our bodies are most apt to burn fat (referred to as the anaerobic threshold). But what the exercise gurus don't realize is that the closer we come to the anaerobic threshold, the further we move away from fat burning. In reality, this benchmark was never intended to measure fat burning. Instead, it was designed for cardiovascular fitness. Training at that heart rate will do wonders for increasing our heart and lung efficiency over time, but it won't do anything for emptying our fat reserves.

If you haven't exercised in a long time or are unaccustomed to this intensity of exercise, the recommended training heart rate noted here will be much too strenuous for your fitness level. Your body won't be able to cope and you will start gasping for air. The minute this happens, the body switches gears and starts burning sugar as its main fuel. If you can't carry on a conversation while exercising without gasping for your next breath, then you are burning sugar instead of fat. Gasping is an indication that there is insufficient oxygen being supplied to the issues. It takes an enormous amount of fuel to burn the dense fat molecules. When there isn't enough oxygen, your body is switching back to third gear (using sugar instead of fat). This is just one reason why people who engage in hour after hour, day after day of strenuous aerobics never ever seem to lose any fat. Imagine all that wasted time and effort!

Body fat is very dense and it requires a great deal of oxygen in order to be burned as fuel.

You're thinking, "If fat needs a lot of oxygen, and we're all gasping for air in aerobics class, aren't we getting a lot of extra oxygen?" Yes and no! The problem is that we can never get enough oxygen when we are overexerting ourselves; that's why we're panting. As the intensity of the activity is increased, the availability of oxygen is actually decreased because we're doing quick, shallow breathing to get air into our lungs, but we're not driving it deep enough. Our bodies have no choice but to switch gears and start mixing more and more sugar into the fuel mix.

The optimal intensity when it comes to fat loss is whatever intensity allows us to take in enough oxygen to burn fat. Usually it is much lower than the proposed anaerobic threshold of 70% and more like 50–60% of maximum heart rate. This is good news for all of you who love taking long walks, an excellent fat-burning exercise.

How Long Do We Have to Work Out?

The length of time we take performing an athletic activity can be just as important as the intensity the exercise is performed at. We can take the intensity down a few speeds to ensure that fat is the primary fuel source used, but how soon do we start using it and, more important, start losing it?

Carmen arrives at the gym and starts her workout with aerobic activity. She punches in her usual 20-minute "fat-burn" routine on her favorite treadmill's computer, and away she goes. Exactly 20 minutes later, she hops off and allows the next confused, over-fat individual his turn. Within minutes she's performing her usual weight-training routine, proud of the fact that she has already taken care of the fat-burning portion of her workout. After all, fat loss is her main objective; muscles can wait. But Carmen, like so many others, is mistaken not only in the duration of the fat-burning portion of her exercise, but also about the order.

What is the optimum duration of cardio for effective fat loss? The answer may be surprising, since the usual limit of time allowed on the cardio equipment is 20 minutes. We've all seen the signs posted in our local gym's cardio theatre: PLEASE RESPECT THE OTHER MEMBERS AND DON'T EXCEED 20 MINUTES ON THE MACHINES. But is 20 minutes enough time to burn fat? The answer, I'm sorry to say, is no!

Starting the Engine: If you live in a cold climate, then your first instinct after your butt hits the cold car seat is to turn on the heat. The problem is that there is no heat to be found; you just started the car, so it will take some time for the engine to warm up. Your body is like that freshly started engine when you begin to exercise—it needs time to warm up.

"High octane" fat fuel is not the starting fuel for cold bodies. The body usually starts warming up with a rich sugar mix instead. In order to change the primary fuel mix to fat, the body must first call into action hormonal and enzymatic responses. Remember: hormones are those tiny, scurrying chemical messengers that give orders to the cells; enzymes are responsible for carrying out the orders. In this case, the adrenal glands start the ball rolling. Stress hormones from these glands that sit atop the kidneys send messages out to the fat cells in order to get them to send some of their fatty acids into the blood. Once these fatty acids are in the bloodstream, they are transported by special carrier proteins to the muscle cells and further escorted into the furnaces of those cells by specific enzymes. This entire response (depending on a host of variables—undigested food, nutrients, etc.) usually takes about 20 minutes to accomplish, which blows apart the theory of burning fat in the first 20 minutes. This means that just around the time we jump off the treadmill, our bodies have switched the fuel mix from sugar to fat. Too bad we're heading for the showers.

Keeping the Engine Revved: There are two things we can do to compensate for the 20-minute start-up for effective fat loss:

- Do the cardio activity longer than 20 minutes to increase the fat-burning effect.
- Do the cardio activity after weight-bearing activity.

Well, the first is a no-brainer. We have already established that effective fat burning begins around the 20-minute mark of cardio exercise, so extending this period would make sense only if fat burning was our goal. But what about the second? Why would performing cardio after weight-bearing exercise help fat loss?

A weight-training routine, performed correctly, is accompanied by a rush at the end of the workout. This "high" feeling comes from a combination of endorphins (pain-desensitizing chemicals that are even more powerful than morphine), anabolic hormones (testosterone and growth hormone) and stress-related chemicals (norepinephrine and epinephrine). Even though we are training primarily in an anaerobic fashion (without oxygen—the first three gears) and utilizing sugar as our main fuel source, we are still invoking a stress response that not only causes that incredible sensation after the exercise, but also frees up those fatty acids.

Doing cardio right after weight training is like getting into a car that has been running for a while. Now all we have to do is turn up the heat, and we will get a blast of warm air. That warm air is a metaphor for our free fatty acids that are now available to be burned through the cardio activity, right from the start. Now we can complete our 20 minutes with the confidence that we have succeeded in burning body fat as our primary fuel source. This is especially true if our muscles have been used regularly and over a long period of time (at least 30 to 45 days) for activities such as progressive resistance training or walking. Conditioned muscles begin to increase their ability to utilize fat as a preferred source of energy.

When Should We Work Out?

Intensity, duration and sequence of exercises ultimately dictate what the fuel mixture will be; it takes 20 minutes to get to the fat-burning phase (a little less if we are conditioned); our bodies can stay in that phase after we've hit the showers. Last question: When is the best time to perform exercise to maximize fat burning? With our metabolic rate being raised for hours afterwards by regular proper exercise, we should reach our fat-loss goals in no time. Well, not exactly. The majority of us perform our exercise in the evenings. This is the time we walk into our local gym and have to take a number just to use the equipment. Exercising in the evening, usually after work, is wrong for two reasons.

- We are usually spent after a day of work and have little energy left for a workout. It's hard enough making dinner after work, let alone training. Our motivation at this time is usually low, and many people will come up with myriad of excuses to avoid training. "I'm too tired, so I'll make up for it tomorrow by doing double." Sure you will, and while you're at it, why don't you complete my workout as well? The scary thing is that the increase in metabolic rate only lasts for the day the exercise is performed (unless you've succeeded in increasing your muscle size). So if we miss a couple of days of exercise, as far as metabolism is concerned, we are right back where we started: fat-land.
- All of that incredible increase in our body's ability to burn fat for hours is shut down by sleep. And even though our sleeping metabolic rate (SMR) may be raised slightly, it hardly makes up for the rate at which we can burn fat while awake.

The best time to exercise for most effective fat-burning potential is first thing in the morning. I know: you barely have enough energy to get out of bed in the morning, let alone hop on a treadmill. Over a short period of time (a few weeks), your body gets used to the new time zone, and before you know it, you can't believe you ever exercised at any other time of day.

Exercising in the morning allows us to take advantage of our body's higher metabolic rate for the entire day. Think about the possibilities. Every time we sit down to eat after exercise is complete, our body will be more efficient at burning the calories from the food. Why would anyone want to lose this advantage by training at night, unless they have no other choice? Besides, the only excuse we have for not training in the morning is because we're too tired. In the morning, gyms aren't nearly as crowded as they are at night. So what's stopping us from training at the most effective time for fat loss?

The Five Muscle-Building, Fat-Burning Exercise Rules

There are right and wrong ways to perform an exercise routine. If you follow the tips presented in this section, I guarantee that progress will be greatly increased. These principles have been gathered from my extensive background in the fitness sciences field.

- Always warm up. A cold muscle is an inactivated muscle. It won't give you much performance, and if you push it too hard, it can be damaged. Always take 10–15 minutes to warm up the body. Walking on a treadmill or peddling on a stationary bike are two good activities that will get the blood pumping. I do not recommend stretching right off the bat since stretching a cold muscle can cause injury to that muscle. If you want to stretch, warm the muscle group first and then stretch.
- Technique is everything, especially when you are weight lifting. If I had a dollar for every time I saw someone training improperly, I'd be a millionaire by now. People seem to be in such a hurry when they work out, lifting weights improperly. Most of the time, these people don't even pay attention to the exercise they are performing. If you want to see results fast, then pay close attention to the way you perform your exercises. Do slow, controlled reps: lift up smoothly and lower the weight to a count of two.
- Don't let your body become bored. Your body adapts to certain exercises rather quickly. If you keep doing the exact same exercises in the same order for any extended period of time (more than a month), your body will adapt and progress will come to an end. You have to keep your nervous system constantly guessing as to what exercises will be performed in what sequence. Research has proven that the body can begin to adapt to the same routine in as little as six sessions.

- There is a distinct, scientifically proven way to perform your set/repetition/intensity range when it comes to effective weight training. Some experts believe that 4–6 reps per exercise builds the most muscle, others believe that 8–10 reps is the best way to go, and still others believe you should strive for 15 and up. All this talk about repetition can be overwhelming to the novice exerciser so in order to understand what a scientifically designed exercise routine should consist of, let's first take a look at the various muscle tissue on the body. You have two kinds of muscles: Type IIa, which are slow-twitch muscle fibers with a high oxidative potential, and Type IIb (best suited for size), which are fast-twitch muscle fibers with a lower oxidative potential.

Type IIa: Slow-twitch muscle fibers use oxygen to produce a steady supply of energy. The fibers function more slowly than their fast-twitch counterparts and are best suited for non-intensive aerobic activities because they do not tire very easily. These muscle fibers have large numbers of capillaries (small blood vessels) that are used to transport oxygen and nutrients into the muscle cells and remove waste products like carbon dioxide. Athletes who excel at endurance activities have a higher percentage of this type of muscle.

Type IIb: Fast-twitch muscles do not have as high a need for oxygen, so they function well in an anaerobic environment. These muscle fibers can contract rapidly, and do very well in high-intensity situations where strength and speed are needed. They are ideally suited for low-endurance activities that require quick bursts of energy, such as weight lifting, sprinting or jumping. They are also called into use during many stop-and-go sports, such as basketball and volleyball. The fast-twitch muscle fibers tire quickly because of the increase in lactic acid, a by-product of low-oxygen (anaerobic) environments. Athletes who excel at short-duration, high-intensity activities seem to have a larger proportion of fast- to slow-twitch muscle fibers.

These different types of fibers in the body require different rep sequences to attain results. Type IIa requires many repetitions for maximum effect and Type IIb requires a low to medium number of repetitions for best results. Perform your exercises varying the rep sequences from 6–15. The exercises could be performed in the following sequence: 1st set: 15 reps; 2nd set: 10 reps; 3rd set: 6–8 reps.

- Always cool down after completion. This is the opportune time to stretch. Take about 10 minutes at the end of the routine and cool down properly. When stretching, make sure you move into the stretch slowly, breathing deeply the entire time. Hold the stretch for at least 10 seconds (preferably 30 seconds to 1 minute) and then slowly come back to the starting position. Most people stretch improperly, which does nothing for the muscle but cause damage. Stretching will also help to remove excess lactic acid that was produced during the weight-training phase of the workout.

HOW MANY CALORIES SHOULD I BURN?

Too many people are much too concerned about the number of calories being burned during their exercise activities. By concentrating our efforts on this aspect of training, it's easy to exercise too long. That's right, we can overdo it just as easily as we can do too little. There comes a time when the positive effects of our physical activities may be negated by the excess production of cortisol, the stress hormone.

We need a little stress to increase the levels of free fatty acids, but too much can cause a drastic increase in cortisol, the muscle-wasting hormone. Dr. Barry Sears, best-selling author of *The Zone* series of books, warns against going over the 45-minute mark when it comes to weight training. Depending on our activity level, soon after 45 minutes the levels of cortisol rise to the point where recovery from the exercise can become blunted. As you recall, cortisol is responsible for stealing valuable nitrogen from muscle tissue and turning the amino acids into sugar in order to create extra energy. The more cortisol is produced, the harder it is to get rid of and the worse off we are for it.

The point is that we will never burn enough calories in the gym to make us happy anyway, but what we may not realize is that the time we spend away from the gym can actually be more beneficial to fat-burning efforts than the time spent doing the actual exercise.

Cardio and weight-bearing activity won't burn a lot of fat during the exercise sessions themselves. The real magic lies in their ability to raise our resting metabolic rate (the rate at which we burn calories at rest) afterwards. A great deal of this post-exercise activity is due to the rise in our anabolic hormones, testosterone and growth hormone approximately 15 minutes after the exercise. As long as we don't blunt this metabolic increase by consuming the wrong foods afterwards, the body will have the ability to burn calories for many hours to come. As a matter of fact, in one study, it was shown that over two-thirds of the fat-burning activity of exercise takes place *after* the actual exercise sessions. This increase in fat-burning potential has been documented at lasting for over 15 hours in highly trained athletes.

When we complete our workout and are either on our way to work, or plopped in front of the TV set watching our favorite programs, our bodies are still at work converting fat into energy. We know this because the post-exercise phase brings with it an increase in resting oxygen consumption and fat-burning enzyme activity. This means that after exercise we have an increased level of fat oxidation and an increased rate of triglyceride fatty acid cycling. Remember how dense the fat is in our cells, and how much oxygen and enzyme activity is needed to annihilate it? Well, this increase in oxygen consumption and enzyme activity after exercise gives us the extra power we need to make this happen. In fact, in repeated blood test studies in Sweden, the fat-burning enzyme (hormone-sensitive lipase) was elevated for a period of 12 hours after a one-hour walk.

Not only can our post-workout time be used for fat burning, we can also burn large amounts of fat while we sleep. The higher the sleeping metabolic rate, the more calories are burned during sleep. Research has proven that exercise can raise our ability to burn fat while sleeping. Exercise can increase our SMR by as much as 18.6%.

BECOMING A GYM RAT OR STAYING HOME GROWN

A health club or gym is a really great place to get physical, but it's not for everyone. The advantages of a gym to some people include the large variety of equipment to choose from; the atmosphere, which can be social and uplifting; and the fact that there is often expert help in the way of a certified trainer to help keep us on the right path. A gym allows the use of a variety of free weights and weight machines that usually aren't available at home. In a gym we can set up a weight circuit, using free weights or plate-loaded machines, which will allow us to move from one exercise to another very efficiently. Also, we can hire a personal trainer for one or more sessions to help us perfect our weight lifting technique. (This will cost some more money, but it may be well worth the price, especially for a novice at weights.)

The downside is that a gym costs money. A gym membership will run anywhere from $35 to $100 a month, and sometimes more for the fancier clubs. In addition, some people feel self-conscious going to a gym—at first glance, it seems that everyone else looks buffed, toned and tanned. It's a little intimidating when Biff, the gym rat, moves into your space and gives you a stare as if to say, "What are *you* doing in my gym?" Also, working out at a gym can take a little more time. There's a drive to get there, the workout, shower and drive home. That can add an extra hour to an already busy day, which might present another excuse for not exercising.

Don't get me wrong. I think the advantages of a gym far outweigh the disadvantages, but the most important thing is to get on the right path to winning the Fat Wars by increasing our level of physical activity any way we can. A word of caution is in order. Do not let a trainer talk you into doing a traditional bodybuilding routine, or, because you are over-fat, recommend that you hit the treadmill for an aerobic blast. The trainer's role should be to just show you the various weight-bearing exercises and how to perform them properly and safely.

While there are virtually dozens of exercises you could do, I prefer the basic lifts—they are easy to do and stimulate the greatest amount of muscle in the least amount of time. As gym memberships go, try to work out a deal with the club. Buy a three-month membership to see if gym training is right for you. Even if you decide to train at home later on, you won't be out a lot of cash.

If you do feel intimidated and self-conscious training at a health club, just remember that others training alongside you will respect you for doing it. They know that what you are trying to accomplish is something that millions of other couch potatoes are avoiding at the same time. No one will make fun of you or condemn you for fighting the good fight. Look around very carefully; there are just as many—if not more—people there who look just like you do. (Where I work out, hard bodies are on the endangered list. The toned, tanned and buffed stand out like sore thumbs because there are so few of them.)

If you can't afford a gym membership, or if you're too intimidated to train with others, or if it takes too much of your time or you just like to train by yourself, then consider training at home or outside. You don't have to use the fancy equipment found in a gym for great results, although I think it helps. You can buy an inexpensive barbell set or a set of adjustable dumbbells from your local mass retailer or sporting goods store for under $60. You can also use other items around your house, such as a towel or a couple of old cans (from soup to paint, as you get more fit) refilled with water or sand.

BE ACTIVE ALL DAY LONG

Every little bit helps. The more active we are throughout the day, the more fat we will burn. Activity increases the body's ability to utilize calories. Every single little thing we take for granted counts. Every time we take the stairs instead of the elevator, every time we choose a parking space a little farther from the mall, and every time we play with our kids instead of saying "I'm too tired" counts! We should not limit activity to formal exercise. While we want fat-burning exercise to be our main means of transformation, other kinds of physical activity will also keep our metabolism high. If we're sitting in front of the television, we can use an elastic band or small weights and just keep moving our muscles under slight resistance. Every little bit helps when we're making progress in the Fat Wars.

FITNESS ON THE GO

If you travel, plan on keeping up with your exercise program while on the road. If you can't get a hotel with a gym, perhaps you can map out a course where you do a variety of exercises, some of which may be with resistance, in an interval fashion.

Special vinyl dumbbells are available that can be filled with water. You can pack them in your suitcase and take them along on your trip, and then fill them up for a quick workout in your hotel room. Elastic bands also can work well (these are what I use when I can't find a gym). Remember: everything counts! A little workout is better than nothing, especially if you are eating out a lot and need to burn the extra calories that restaurant food typically contains. (You could always leave some of it on the plate.)

If you truly want to lose fat and keep it off for life, you know what has to be done. Regular exercise is definitely the smart way toward permanent fat loss, but there are some specific ground rules that can lead to success or failure. Here they are:

- Don't expect to transform your body overnight. We seem to forget the road that got us here in the first place. We didn't wake up one morning to suddenly discover layers of fat on our buff physiques. We got here one Twinkie and one sedentary day at a time. It all adds up. Since you didn't become fat overnight, don't expect to lose all your fat overnight. Give yourself sufficient time to reach your goals, an ounce of fat at a time.

- What you did in the past doesn't count. You may be skeptical that this new information on exercise will work for you. You may have tried physical activity before, only to see no results and drop out. The improvements just weren't worth the effort. That's all about to change. If applied correctly, you will lose fat and lots of it. This means everyone—men, women and children—regardless of how over-fat they are.

- Get into the Do Zone. The words on these pages will not burn your fat. *You* will burn your fat. You must become self-motivated to succeed. The best way to get into the habit of regular exercise is through plenty of practice, beginning with the exercises outlined in the *Fat Wars* 45-Day Transformation Plan in Chapter 14.

- Take an honest look at the reasons why you (and not your situation) stop yourself from exercising. Don't beat yourself up for not getting physically active. There will be times that are out of your control when you won't be able to exercise. More often than not, a block in training is just in your mind. Don't put off exercise for one more minute; as the Nike ads say, "Just Do It!"

Apply the strategies you've learned here as if they were the last detail to your fat-loss battle plan because they are. Without exercise, you will fall short of your objectives. And even if you lose weight, you will likely gain it all back, and then some. Is that what you really want? Or would you rather lose the fat weight and keep it off permanently? I thought so.

14

The *Fat Wars*
Action Plan

This chapter is designed to help you develop your personal *Fat Wars* 45-Day Transformation Plan. Why 45 days to transformation? From experience, it generally takes at least 45 days to notice a significant change in how you look, feel and perform. Remember: this is not a get-lean-quick scheme! It takes dedication and hard work to change a lifestyle that has probably been with you for a very long time. Nothing happens overnight; it takes numerous small steps to accomplish something as important as life transformation.

In this plan, 45 days to transformation really means nine weeks—the plan is broken up into nine, five-day cycles starting on Monday and ending on Friday. This does not mean that on the weekends you can forget all the changes you've made and start back at square one on Monday. Instead, the five-day cycles are designed to give your body a chance to adapt to the stimulus of the resistance and cardio exercises as well as the new way of eating. You can choose to continue your aerobic exercise in the form of walking or some other low-impact activity on the weekends, or you can choose to take a break from any exercise; it's really up to you. Listen to your body—sometimes it will want a rest to recover from a tough week; sometimes you will want to get out there and play. Whatever you choose, it is very important to stay close to your new eating strategy throughout the nine weeks (yes, this means weekends, too).

Make a genuine commitment to nine weeks. Forty-five days is not that long a period to establish new habits for a healthier, fitter future. I have seen many people reluctantly begin the transformation period of the *Fat Wars*

Plan only to say how glad they were that they stuck to it, and how quickly the time passed. The way you will feel at the end of the first 45 days will amaze you, not to mention those around you. It's a small, new beginning that may not seem significant at the time, but in the long run, you will change your life as well as your body.

The following quote from an on-line book called *Life's Riddle* by Nils A. Amneus sums up the philosophy for change here:

> ***Every Effort Counts***
> *A stone placed on one pan of a scale may keep this down for a long time, but a fine trickle of sand continuously pouring on the other pan will in time balance and then outweigh the stone. In the beginning it seemed as though the sand had no effect for the stone remained unmoved, then, suddenly, it is lifted. And so it is with our own actions. We do not know how big our "stone," our accumulation of demerit, may be, and we may have to wait a long time before the results of our efforts will become apparent. But as every grain of sand did its part towards outweighing the stone, so every effort at self-improvement, even the smallest, counts, and if continued, the time will come when all demerit will be balanced.*

Your stone can be viewed as your excess body fat, and the sand as the little changes you make every day during the 45-day transformation period. Before you know it, the stone has been lifted and you are a new, improved version of your former self. But once the excess fat has been lifted, you must maintain your new lifestyle changes so that the fat never returns. This is why you must remain committed to your new lifestyle and never look back. Luckily, good health is addictive.

THE BEST TIME TO CHANGE

Fat Wars was written to give you a scientific approach to change the way you look, feel and perform. It is in your best interest not to put off this change any longer—start changing your habits today. Change is one of the hardest things to accomplish; it's hard to break out of old habits that we are used to. We all get caught up in our own little comfort zones because they are familiar, even though poor health habits have gotten us where we are today.

Failure, believe it or not, can also be something we are the most comfortable with. If you have been overweight most of your life, even though you may want to change on some level (probably a very deep one), being overweight may be the state in which you are the most comfortable. This comfort zone (snug in your protective coating of fat) allows you to deal with situations you are most familiar with. If you were to shed this protective layer, you would be on unfamiliar ground; you would look, feel and perform differently—better—than you ever dreamed. Instead of seeing this as a scary prospect, accept that it will be an exciting one.

THE *FAT WARS* 45-DAY TRANSFORMATION PLAN

During the first 45 days of the rest of your life, there will be some positive changes to set the stage for permanent fat loss. Cell sensitivity to insulin will increase, reducing resting insulin levels, blood fats and glucose. This will make your muscle cells happy and ready to work for you by burning fat.

During the 45-day period your body will become accustomed to the resistance and aerobic portions of the exercise component, and muscle growth will occur. In men, this will be an increase in muscle mass and strength, as well as an increase in transport proteins, fat-burning enzymes and immune factors. Women will also experience an increase in strength and intracellular proteins, but without the bulk gains that men experience. Levels of cortisol (the muscle-wasting hormone) will begin to drop and levels of glucagon (the fat-releasing hormone) will rise. While you will burn fat, remember that you will be building muscle, which weighs more. Look for a leaner you, but not necessarily a lighter one.

Don't become discouraged in the first few weeks—you are bound to lose some battles along the road toward mastering fat loss. Your body has become accustomed to the extra fat that covers the lean you underneath, so at first it may be reluctant to change. Just keep on plugging away and in 45 days you will be amazed at your progress.

Make a full commitment to yourself to complete the *Fat Wars* 45-Day Transformation Plan and to stick to the recommendations as closely as possible. Take stock of what you're eating now and how to change it. Make a commitment to assess your diet and start to buy and eat more healthy food, five or six times a day. Take a step-by-step approach to making these new improved habits part of your life.

The Importance of Water

When it comes to increasing our overall health profile, we often forget to increase our consumption of one of the most important elements of all—water. Water is essential to the biochemical functions of the human body (we are, in fact, mostly water!). Your bones are one-quarter water. Your brain and muscles are three-quarters water. Your blood and lungs are over 80% water. Next to oxygen, water is the most important ingredient for sustaining life. Then why don't the majority of us drink enough of it?

Well, you might say, "I drink plenty of liquid: juice, coffee, tea, sodas." Nothing can take the place of water. Many of us may indeed be dehydrated and not even know it!

During exercise, it's imperative to increase your water intake because water is vital in cardiovascular function and temperature regulation. As you exercise, your muscles create a lot of extra heat. The heat is transported through tiny blood vessels called capillaries near the surface of your skin. The release of perspiration from your sweat glands and its evaporation has a cooling effect on the skin as well as the blood in the capillaries beneath it.

Sweating is an essential mechanism in your body's cooling system and if your body doesn't have enough water to make this system run smoothly, your blood-carrying capacity diminishes. Don't forget: it is the blood's role to carry nutrients such as oxygen, glucose, fatty acids and proteins to the muscles to create energy. The blood must also remove the toxic residue of metabolism, such as carbon dioxide and lactic acid. Since your circulatory system is almost 70% water, the extra demand for water can be quite severe. Intensive exercise can cause a person to lose 5–8 lbs. of fluid through perspiration, evaporation and exhalation. Studies show that for every pound of fluid lost, there is a significant drop in the efficiency with which the body produces energy. Try to consume clean filtered water throughout the day.

Losing excess fat can also cause a release of toxins into your body since many toxins become lodged in the fatty tissue. Water is essential in the detoxification process, and since you will be dropping fat, you will need all you can drink.

In his best-selling book, *Your Body's Many Cries for Water,* Dr. Fereydoon Batmanghelidj suggests that somewhere during our evolution, the signals for thirst and hunger may have become the same. Dr. Batmanghelidj believes that often when we think we are hungry, we are in fact just thirsty. So in order to cut down on the impulse to overeat, it is recommended that you drink a glass of water before eating. This way, you will be guaranteed not to overeat to satisfy an urge for water intake. Carry your water with you everywhere you go (I even bring my water to bed) in a closed container, and drink it through a straw to avoid swallowing excess air.

You have learned what type of exercises to perform and how to do them for maximum effect. Now's the time to put this into action. If you have never trained with weights before, it would be a good idea to hire a personal trainer to take you through the first week of the *Fat Wars* 45-Day Transformation Plan. Please stick closely to these exercises and their format. The routine was designed to make sure that you see results within the 45 days.

The supplements recommended in this book can be added at any time during the plan, but it's best if they are included right from the start. Furthermore, this plan was not designed to cause you to burn out, so don't burn the candle at both ends. Get plenty of rest and allow yourself enough time for deep sleep to restore your body so that you can continue to progress. Don't forget that rest gives your body a chance to rebuild itself. Remember—after the first 45 days, you won't want to look back! Follow this step-by-step strategy and say hello to the new you!

CRAFTING YOUR *FAT WARS* FOOD PLAN

How Much Can You Eat in a Day?

For best results on the *Fat Wars* 45-Day Transformation Plan, you will have to figure out your total daily calorie allotment. Remember that if you take in more calories than you burn throughout the day, the rest will end up as winter insulation.

Quick Method: Use this if you don't have access to a body mass analyzer. Multiply your weight in pounds by the appropriate number below:

- Sedentary woman: 12; Sedentary man: 14
- Active woman: 15; Active man: 17

The result is a rough estimate of your daily calorie allotment. This is not as exact a measurement as the one recommended below, but it will definitely get you started on your fat-loss path until you can get your body fat percentage measured by a more precise means.

Since your goal is to lose fat, you should subtract 500 calories from your daily calorie allotment (at the same time, you will be increasing your daily activity level). This should result in the loss of approximately 2 lbs. of fat per week, which is the healthiest way to permanent fat loss, according to research. Using the example of a soon-to-be-active woman who presently weighs 180 lbs., the equation would look like this: $180 \times 15 = 2{,}700$ calories (minus 500 calories for fat loss) equals a daily calorie intake of 2,200 calories.

If you find that your fat is not melting away fast enough (be reasonable here), you can adjust your daily calorie intake by lowering it by no more than 250 calories at a time until you notice the fat coming off again. Do not lower your daily calories more than once a week. If you subtracted 250 calories from your daily allotment, stay at this new calorie intake for the whole week.

Total Calories, Using a Body Mass Analyzer

If you have access to a body mass analyzer, then follow these recommendations:

- *Step 1:* To calculate your lean body weight measurement, you must first get your body-fat percentage tested using one of the tests recommended in Appendix I. To find out your lean body weight measurement (the total amount of lean tissue, excluding fat, your body is carrying), you multiply your current weight by the body-fat percentage revealed by the test. For instance, if you are a woman who presently weighs 180 lbs. and the test showed you have a body-fat percentage of 40, your lean body weight is the remaining 60%, or 108 lbs. Since the ideal body-fat percentage for a man is 15 and for a woman is 24, you multiply your lean body weight by one of these percentages (or whatever percentage you are striving for). For a body-fat percentage of 24, this woman would multiply 108 (her lean body weight) by 24% and add the result (26 lbs.) to her lean body weight; this will tell her that her ideal weight is 134 lbs. Now she knows that she is approximately 46 lbs. from her ideal body weight.
- *Step 2:* Now, take the new ideal weight (in the above example, 134 lbs.) and multiply it by 10. Here, the equation would be: $134 \times 10 = 1,340$.
- Step 3: Using the chart below, multiply your present weight by the appropriate activity factor. Using the example above, the woman who weighs 180 lbs. and leads a very active life (especially with her new *Fat Wars* exercise plan) would use $180 \times 7 = 1,260$.

ENERGY ACTIVITY CHART

Sedentary	Active	Very Active	Extremely Active
3	5	7	10

- *Step 4:* Your calorie maintenance level is the total of the two calculations from steps 2 and 3. Using our example above, the equation would be $1,340 + 1,260 = 2,600$ calories per day for maintenance.

- *Step 5:* Since your goal is to lose fat, you should again subtract 500 calories from your daily calorie allotment, all the while increasing your daily activity level. This should again result in the loss of approximately 2 lbs. of fat per week. Using the above example, 2,600 calories minus 500 equals a daily calorie intake of 2,100.

Again, if you find that the fat is not melting away fast enough, you can adjust your daily calorie intake by lowering it by about 250 calories at a time, but no more than once a week.

Finding Your Macronutrient Meal Profile

Now that you have calculated your daily calorie intake, you need to work out your macronutrient meal profile: the amount of carbohydrates, dietary fats and dietary proteins you should have at any one meal. As discussed in Chapter 11, the macronutrient profile that has been found to be most effective for long-term fat loss is the 40% carbohydrates, 30% dietary fats and 30% dietary proteins profile. Please refer to Chapters 6, 7 and 8 for a quick review of the types of foods for each macronutrient. To figure out the equation for your macronutrient meal profile, follow the next steps.

Total Calories per day, based on your present weight, activity level and fat loss goals	Multiply by:	Divide by the number of calories per gram:	Divide by number of meals per day (adjust to your own requirements)	Macronutrient Profile
	.40	4	4	____ g carbohydrates per meal
	.30	9	4	____ g dietary fat per meal
	.30	4	4	____ g dietary protein per meal

For example, our 180 lb. woman has used the quick method to calculate that her daily calorie intake should be 2,200 to achieve her fat loss goals. She is going to have six meals a day. Her chart will look like this:

Total Calories	Multiply by:	Divide by calories per gram:	Divide by Number of Meals:	Macronutrient Profile
2,200	.40	4	6	37 g carbohydrates per meal
2,200	.30	9	6	12 g dietary fat per meal
2,200	.30	4	6	27.5 g dietary protein per meal

As mentioned in chapter 11, The Fat Wars Eating Principles, the final meal of the day (meal 5 or 6) should be adjusted to contain as little carbohydrate source as possible (preferably none). The reason for this adjustment in the evening is to allow for effective fat burning through maximum growth hormone release due to lowered insulin levels. This is the only meal that requires this adjustment, all the others should remain as close as possible to the 40-30-30 principle.

No Wheat, No Rice
For best results during the *Fat Wars* 45-Day Transformation Plan, it is important to avoid wheat and rice of any kind. This means that for the duration of the nine weeks, no bread (the only exception being bread that comes from sprouted grain and contains no gluten), no pasta and no rice. These are the carbohydrate sources that seem to cause the greatest insulin spikes and cravings for sugar, so avoiding them will make things much easier. After the nine weeks, you can reintroduce them into your diet; once again the choice is yours.

PUTTING YOUR EXERCISE PLAN TOGETHER
This part of the transformation plan is key to your success, since this is how you will increase your body's ability to burn fat. This exercise component is based on the periodization philosophy of resistance training, which other trainers and I have used with great success for fat loss. The routines are progressively changed for maximized benefits. There are also two different programs of routines for you to do once you establish your exercise habit. The first one consists of three resistance training sessions per week (Monday, Wednesday and Friday); each session includes routines that work the muscles all over your body.

The second program changes to a split routine, which involves resist-ance training four times a week; in this program you work two separate groups of muscles in your body twice a week each, for a total of four train-ing sessions during these weeks. The weekends are always considered an option for aerobic activity during the transformation period, but it is highly recommended that you remain very active on the off days of the resistance portion of the program, which also includes weekends.

When exercising, there is a target heart rate range you should be aiming for to maximize fat burning. The goal is to keep your system from running out of oxygen and switching to sugar for fuel instead of fat. Calculate your target heart rate during the exercise program, using 50–60% of (220 minus your age) as a good target heart rate for optimum fat loss. As an example, if you are 40 years old, you would subtract 40 from 220 to get 180; 50–60% of 180 gives you a training intensity level of 90–108 beats per minute. You should start out at the lower percentage, which is 50%, and increase the percentage as you get in better shape.

Establishing Your Heart Rate: There are a couple of ways to measure your heart rate. One is accomplished manually, and the other requires a mechanical device that takes regular measurements of your pulse.

1. *Manual Method:* There are two areas on your body where you can get a good pulse read; one is on your wrist and the other is on your neck.
   - On the underside of your wrist, locate the tendon that runs from the forearm to the hand. Next, using the index and middle fingers of the opposite hand, press the thumb side of that tendon just below your hand. You should feel your radial pulse.
   - You can also feel your pulse by locating your carotid artery on your neck. Place your index and middle fingers just below your jaw (on the same side as your hand). Feel around for a slight indentation and keep your fingers gently pressed on that spot until you feel your pulse.
   - Once you have located your pulse in either spot, count the beats for one full minute. *Voila,* that's your heart rate.

2. *Mechanical Method:* There are many heart-rate monitors available on the market that automatically measure your heart rate throughout your exercise activity. If you can afford a quality device, it is a very practical tool for staying within your target heart rate. The brand names I recommend are listed in Appendix I.

> ### *Exercising Safely*
> Since *Fat Wars* is not intended to be an exercise manual, but instead offers a suggested exercise protocol to get you started on your successful fat-burning way, you should enlist the aid of a qualified personal trainer to ensure that you do the resistance exercises properly and safely. If you do not want to do this, or can't afford the services of a trainer, then I recommend that you purchase a book on resistance training that has easy-to-follow diagrams of each exercise. One recommended title is *Weight Training for Dummies* by Suzanne Schlosberg and Liz Neporent.
>
> If you have any physical limitations, joint pains, chronic muscle aches, or if you experience sudden or recurring dizziness at any time during your exercises, you must check with your health care provider before continuing. (If you haven't been active for some time, it is advisable to check with your health care provider before you start.)

WEEK 1

Use this week to ease into your new lifestyle commitments. If you are not familiar with stretching movements, use this time to find a qualified fitness trainer who can take you through the routine until you can do them easily.

Monday to Friday:	
Warm-up	5 minutes of slow walking
Resistance training	none
Aerobic exercise	Take a 1-hour walk every day this week (preferably first thing in the morning on an empty stomach). When you are walking, be aware of your posture: your chin should be held high and your back should be straight. Swing your arms. Get your whole body into the walk. There should be a good amount of deep breathing, but not so much that you are gasping for air—you should be able to carry on a conversation.
Abdominal crunches	3 sets of abdominal crunches following each walk. Start with sets of 5 repetitions (reps).
Cool down	stretch for about 10 minutes

> ### *Instructions for Proper Abdominal Crunches*
> - Lie flat on your back with your knees bent and your feet together flat on the floor. Your feet should be about 10–15 inches from your buttocks.
> - Your hands should be crossed on your chest, by your side or cupped behind your ears.
> - Without moving your lower body, curl your upper torso up and in toward your knees, until your shoulder blades are as high off the ground as you can get them. Only your shoulder blades should lift—not your lower back.
> - As you come to the highest point, tighten and flex your abdominals for a second.
> - Slowly lower yourself back to the starting position.
>
> **Cautions:**
> - Don't jerk yourself up to achieve the exercise. Slowly bring yourself up using only your abdominal muscles.
> - Don't let your lower back rise off the floor. Go up until you feel your abdominals become tight; hold the position for a second.
> - Don't move quickly. You must do this exercise very slowly and resist on the way back down.

WEEK 2

Add a routine of eight resistance exercises on Monday, Wednesday and Friday of this week. Use dumbbells for all the exercises listed, in order to stimulate the best muscle contractions.

Follow the recommended rep schemes presented here. If a specified rep scheme calls for 20 repetitions per set, it is important to the outcome of the set that you perform only the set number of reps (in this case, 20). If your specified rep scheme is 20 reps per set, then by your nineteenth rep, you should be barely able to complete the final one. Pick a weight for the specified exercise that you can only perform the recommended number of repetitions with. When you are able to do more than the recommended number of reps, it is time to increase the size of the weight. (Consult a personal trainer, weight-training book or www.fatwars.com if you are unsure of how to choose proper weights.)

Perform one set of 20 repetitions for each exercise, with a 1-minute rest between sets.

Monday, Wednesday and Friday:

Warm-up	10 minutes of walking or riding a bike to increase the blood flow		
Resistance training	*Exercises* *Repetitions*	*Sets*	
	Dumbbell Squats (thighs)	1	20
	Dumbbell Stiff-Legged Dead-Lift (rear of thigh)	1	20
	Dumbbell Bench-Press (chest)	1	20
	Dumbbell Rows (back)	1	20
	Dumbbell Side Laterals (shoulders)	1	20
	Dumbbell Curls (biceps)	1	20
	Dumbbell Tricep Extension (triceps)	1	20
	Standing Calf Raises (calves)	1	20
Aerobic exercise	Walk for 30 minutes at your target heart rate. Warm up and cool down for about 5 minutes at a slower pace.		
Abdominal crunches	3 sets of abdominal crunches following each walk. Do 10 reps in each set.		
Cool down	stretch for about 10 minutes		

Tuesday and Thursday:

Warm-up	5 minutes of slow walking
Resistance training	None
Aerobic exercise	30–60 minutes of walking
Abdominal crunches	3 sets of abdominal crunches following each walk. Do 10 reps in each set.
Cool down	stretch for about 10 minutes

WEEKS 3 and 4

You will be staying with the same weight for both sets in your resistance training program. Since your muscles will be fatiguing on each consecutive set, don't be surprised if you have trouble doing the 20 repetitions on the second set. Do as many as you can (try your best to get 20 reps).

Monday, Wednesday and Friday:

Warm-up	10 minutes of walking or riding a bike to increase the blood flow		
Resistance training	*Exercises*	*Sets*	
	Repetitions		
	Dumbbell Squats (thighs)	2	20
	Dumbbell Stiff-Legged Dead-Lift (rear of thigh)	2	20
	Dumbbell Bench-Press (chest)	2	20
	Dumbbell Rows (back)	2	20
	Dumbbell Side Laterals (shoulders)	2	20
	Dumbbell Curls (biceps)	2	20
	Dumbbell Tricep Extension (triceps)	2	20
	Standing Calf Raises (calves)	2	20
Aerobic exercise	Walk for 30 minutes at your target heart rate. Warm up and cool down at a slower pace.		
Abdominal crunches	3 sets of abdominal crunches following each walk. Do 15 reps in each set.		
Cool down	stretch for about 10 minutes		

Tuesday and Thursday:

Warm-up	5 minutes of slow walking
Resistance training	None
Aerobic exercise	30–60 minutes of walking
Abdominal crunches	3 sets of abdominal crunches following each walk. Do 15 reps in each set.
Cool down	stretch for about 10 minutes

WEEK 5

The number of sets per resistance training exercise will increase from 2 to 3. The number of repetitions in each set will change from 20 to 15. Monday and Friday workouts will be at full force, but on Wednesday, ease up on your training intensity (i.e., use a lighter weight), moving through each exercise with as little rest as possible (1 minute, max.). Although the weights can be eased up a bit on Wednesday, the repetitions stay the same, allowing for an easier workout.

On each day, stay with the same weight for all 3 sets. Since your muscles will be fatiguing on each consecutive set, don't be surprised if you have trouble doing the 15 repetitions on the second and third set. Do as many as you can (try your best to get 15 reps).

Monday, Wednesday and Friday:

Warm-up	10 minutes of walking or riding a bike to increase the blood flow		
Resistance training	*Exercises* *Repetitions*		*Sets*
	Dumbbell Squats (thighs)	3	15
	Dumbbell Stiff-Legged Dead-Lift (rear of thigh)	3	15
	Dumbbell Bench-Press (chest)	3	15
	Dumbbell Rows (back)	3	15
	Dumbbell Side Laterals (shoulders)	3	15
	Dumbbell Curls (biceps)	3	15
	Dumbbell Tricep Extension (triceps)	3	15
	Standing Calf Raises (calves)	3	15
Aerobic exercise	Walk for 30 minutes at your target heart rate. Warm up and cool down at a slower pace.		
Abdominal crunches	3 sets of abdominal crunches following each walk. (20 reps per set)		
Cool down	stretch for about 10 minutes		

Tuesday and Thursday:

Warm-up	5 minutes of slow walking
Resistance training	None
Aerobic exercise	30–60 minutes of walking
Abdominal crunches	3 sets of abdominal crunches following each walk. (20 reps per set)
Cool down	stretch for about 10 minutes

WEEKS 6 to 9

Now that your metabolism has been jump-started and your body has adapted to the weight training from the previous month, your workout format will change to the split routine. Instead of repeating the same training session to work all muscle groups, you will now use two different training sessions that target two different sets of muscle groups. This new split routine will allow some muscle groups to gain extra rest (for recuperation) while others are being trained. During these weeks, you will train with weights on Monday and Tuesday, and then again on Thursday and Friday.

You will now perform two exercises for each muscle group instead of one. Up until this point in your transformation program, you have been performing compound exercises, which are exercises that use a number of muscle groups. The split routines incorporate both a compound exercise and an isolation exercise. Unlike compound exercises, isolation exercises work only a single muscle or a specific group of muscles.

You will also add a barbell exercise into this part of your transformation routine. There are 3 sets in the first exercise for each muscle group, followed by 2 sets for the second exercise (isolation), for a total of 5 sets per body part. Certain smaller muscle groups (such as arms) will only require 3 sets of one exercise in total. The repetitions per exercise will be 10–12. This will allow for heavier weights than previously used for increased muscle strength, size and function.

Follow this routine for the remainder of the nine weeks.

Monday and Friday:			
Warm-up	10 minutes of walking or riding a bike to increase the blood flow		
Resistance training	*Exercises* *Repetitions*	*Sets*	
	Barbell Squats (thighs)	3	10–12
	Seated Leg Extensions	2	10–12
	Stiff-Legged Dead-Lift (rear of thigh)	3	10–12
	Lying Leg Curls	2	10–12
	Side Laterals (shoulders)	3	10–12
	Calf Raises (calves)	3	10–12
Aerobic exercise	Walk for 20 minutes at your target heart rate. Warm up and cool down at a slower pace.		
Abdominal crunches	3 sets of abdominal crunches following each walk. (25 reps per set)		
Cool down	stretch for about 10 minutes		

Tuesday and Thursday:

Warm-up	10 minutes of walking or riding a bike to increase the blood flow		
Resistance training	*Exercises* *Repetitions*	*Sets*	
	Bench-Press	3	10–12
	Incline Press	2	10–12
	Bent-Over Rows	3	10–12
	Seated Cable Rows	2	10–12
	Standing Barbell Curls (biceps)	3	10–12
	Barbell Tricep Extension (triceps)	3	10–12
Aerobic exercise	Walk for 20 minutes at your target heart rate. Warm up and cool down at a slower pace.		
Abdominal crunches	3 sets of abdominal crunches following each walk. (25 reps per set)		
Cool down	stretch for about 10 minutes		

Wednesday:

Warm-up	5 minutes of slow walking
Resistance training	None
Aerobic exercise	30–60 minutes of walking
Abdominal crunches	3 sets of abdominal crunches following each walk. (25 reps per set)
Cool down	stretch for about 10 minutes

After the 45-Day Transformation Period

If you stick with the advice in this section, you will be successful in achieving your *Fat Wars* goal. Once the 45-day transformation period is over, your new life will be just beginning. All the workout suggestions have been based on a scientific approach to progressive resistance using a periodization training philosophy. The periodization philosophy allows for three four-month cycles of various training routines to be performed in any given year. This type of training allows for constant improvement in all areas of athleticism.

Periodization Training

Periodization training is a definition for any training plan that changes your workouts at regular intervals. It involves changing many variables pertaining to a workout routine, including the number of repetitions in a set, the kind of exercises performed, the amount of weight used and the amount of time allowed for rest in between your sets. It is a scientifically sound way to ensure continual improvements and not hit the all-too-common training plateau, where at a certain time in one's training cycle, all progress seems to come to an abrupt halt.

Periodization training includes cycles of both intense and less intense training periods throughout the year so that you reduce long intervals of stress on your body. When people train the conventional way, they sometimes accumulate stress to the point of doing damage. By alternating intense and less intense workout cycles, muscle strain and training plateaus are prevented. A typical periodization plan will consist of three four-month cycles. Each month would allow for a new set of training rules, for instance:

- The first month may dictate a high-rep scheme of 20 reps per set but only 1 or 2 sets per exercise. Therefore you would be lifting relatively light weights (low intensity).
- The second month may consist of a lower rep scheme of 12–15 reps per set with perhaps 2–3 sets per exercise, allowing you to lift slightly heavier weights (higher intensity).
- The third month would call for still a lower rep scheme of 8–10 reps per set and 3–4 sets per exercise, allowing for relatively heavy weights to increase strength and size (intense).
- The final month (month 4) would be the most intense, using the lowest rep scheme of 4–6 reps per set and 3–5 sets per exercise, allowing for the heaviest weights used in the four months, which would further increase the strength of the muscle fibers.

After the fourth month of training, begin the routine again at the first month to allow for maximum recovery and recuperation from the more intense month of the routine. There are three of these cycles in a typical year. Of course, this is just a very generalized outlook on the principles of periodization training, but enough to give you some insight into its principles. For a detailed approach to this training method, you should read *Periodization Breakthrough* by Dr. Steven Fleck and Dr. William Kraemer.

The routines presented in the *Fat Wars* 45-Day Transformation Plan will bring you through two of these periodization cycles of four weeks in length. The goal of this transformation plan is an increase in both muscle size and fat-burning activity. The basic periodization goal per cycle is to progress from high-volume (higher reps/sets), low-intensity (lighter weights) through the first two cycles to low-volume (lower reps/sets) and high-intensity (heavier weights) training through the final two cycles. As you continue on your new life-path (and I know you will), you should complete the last two cycles of a properly designed training program by progressively lowering the repetitions of the exercises performed while increasing the weights used. (Please refer to a well-designed training manual or a qualified personal trainer versed in periodization training). Cardio activity should remain constant throughout the various cycles. This way your body will continue to progress and avoid any plateaus.

Creatine Monohydrate, the Exercise Supplement

Once you start your exercise program, if you are having trouble adapting to the resistance exercise or want to increase the effectiveness of your recovery time between workouts, you can try a supplement called creatine.

Creatine is an important part of cell energetics that combines with phosphates to make phosphocreatine (PC). PC replenishes lost, energy-rich phosphates that are used to make adenosine triphosphate (ATP), your cell's main energy currency. Creatine has been shown in many studies to increase muscle power in speed/strength athletes like football players, sprinters and weight lifters. Research also shows that creatine has a pronounced anabolic effect by helping to increase protein synthesis in trained muscles.

Creatine can increase fat-loss results when accompanied by a proper weight-training routine. Creatine helps the muscles work harder and recuperate faster by replenishing energy and stimulating muscle growth. Many research studies have given subjects 5 g four or five times daily for five to seven days. Recent research shows that we don't need this much creatine, nor do we need to load it as long as we have been.

Five grams three times a day for three or four days should be sufficient to start with. This is considered a loading phase and is designed to saturate the muscles with a lot of creatine. After the loading period, the daily dose is reduced to 5 g per day, usually taken postexercise.

You do not have to load creatine. Instead you can take a dose of 4–5 g daily over several weeks. This works well and allows the muscle (and intracellular proteins) to recover from training and grow even faster. The most common and affordable form of creatine is creatine monohydrate. You may notice a slight weight gain from creatine monohydrate during the first two weeks of use. This is because creatine helps to swell cells by increasing their water content. Don't worry, the extra water weight is a temporary phenomenon that is actually helpful in increasing the cell's anabolic activity. Creatine is very safe and there have been no reported adverse effects to its long-term use, even at higher doses. It is best absorbed when mixed with a high-glycemic carbohydrate shake after training (see Chapter 11).

Creatine works especially well when combined with the amino acids glutamine and taurine. You can purchase creatine as a pure powder, or combined with other nutrients in a powder beverage. Either way, a 2–5 g dose once daily after training should help your exercising efforts.

THE FIVE KEYS TO REACHING YOUR FAT-LOSS GOAL

1: Visualize Your Goal

In order to achieve, you must really believe, and in order to believe, you must first visualize the goal. The first step in achieving your goal is this one.

- *Be as detailed as possible when you visualize.* Picture yourself in your new body and lifestyle. How do you look in your new body? What do you feel like? How are people around you responding? How confident do you feel? How energized are you? Whatever you really want to look like, picture it as if it has already happened.
- *Take a picture of yourself wearing a bathing suit.* Place it where you will be able to see it often. Nothing motivates people more than being reminded of how they looked before they started. Whenever you feel like going off your plan, look at the picture and visualize your new body.
- *Believe it.* It's like acting in a sense; you need to play the part of the person you want to become. No matter what happens between now and the day you want to achieve your goal, in your mind, you have already achieved it. This way, you have already accepted the reality of the new you.

2: Write Down Your Fat-Loss Goal

Be specific, but also be realistic when it comes to the time frame for achieving your goal. For instance, if you presently register 40% body fat but your goal is to be at 24%, don't expect to reach your goal in a month's time. (Note that you're not setting a target for weight loss in pounds—the leaner you will be adding fat-burning muscle.) Be honest with yourself—don't set yourself up for failure. Write down achievable time lines for your objective: the first three weeks, the second three weeks, and beyond. Your goal for the first three weeks could be to get your new routines in place; by six weeks you aim to lose 3–4% body fat. Be specific with dates. Don't just say "in three weeks." Write down the actual date three, six, nine weeks from when you start.

Identify the whys of your goal, for instance, "I want to lose 3–4% body fat by November 30 because I'm going to Hawaii and I want to look good. I also want to lose this fat because I know that I will feel better about myself and have more energy to enjoy my trip. Once I feel better, I will continue to work toward the healthy state I always knew I could achieve. My health is really what matters most to me. Losing this weight is only the beginning of a whole new me." It is always important to be as specific as possible when you write these goals.

Once you've told yourself what you're doing and why, let others know what you are doing. You must be sincere about this step: if you jokingly say, "You won't recognize me next summer," then even you won't take it seriously. Be strong in your conviction. Trust me, there is no better way to guarantee success than by putting extra pressure on yourself by letting your friends know what you are striving for. Don't be afraid to ask for their support. Believe me, they will be the first to let you know if you're not sticking to your plan.

3: Write Down How You're Going to Reach Your Goal

In order to follow the *Fat Wars* 45-Day Transformation Plan, you will have to make some changes. Let's be realistic here, you have developed— how shall we say?—some bad habits along the way that got you where you are today. Many of them have to go: how about those late nights that deprive you of badly needed sleep? That one positive change will mean that you will be able to wake up one hour earlier each day and you'll have time to complete the energizing exercise portion of the plan.

You will also have to assess what you've been eating, plan the changes that will help you burn fat, and eliminate many of what you have come to rely on as "comfort foods." (You know what these are.) Write down everything you can think of that needs to be changed to guarantee success. If you've never tried anything like this before, the changes will feel dramatic—but so will the emerging new you. If you've tried lots of diets before and you've been exercising, it will be a matter of making adjustments. Remember, after 45 days, you'll feel so great that no one will have to convince you to continue.

4: Keep a Log of Your Progress

It's time to take charge of your success. Remove all the guesswork and chaos from your training and diet program by keeping an accurate record of each workout and each day's food intake. Most of the people who fail to reach their fat-loss goals tried to follow a routine intuitively. Winning your personal Fat War requires careful planning and organization, the setting of priorities (the new you) and the willingness to spend some time tracking your changes (or lack of them).

If you are willing to keep a log of your training and diet activities, then you will have a precise record of what works best for you and how much you've really changed. You can use the sample charts shown here to get you started. A training journal will help you:

- see progress from each workout
- know how many repetitions you performed and how much weight you used in your last workout
- have an accurate record of exercises or a routine that worked for you
- have an accurate record of exercises or a routine that didn't work for you
- know when to make adjustments in your training cycles

A diet journal will help you:

- keep track of how many calories you are taking in
- keep an accurate record of the best calorie intake for your needs
- ensure that you are within your proper macronutrient profile
- know when to make adjustments in your food intake

Fat Wars Training Log   *Week of :*

Warm-up

Resistance training	Exercises	Sets	Weight	Repetitions

Aerobic
exercise

Abdominal
crunches

Cool down

Comments/
Dates
Performed

Log into www.fatwars.com <http://www.fatwars.com>, and get the latest up-to-date information on fat burning meal plans, shake recipes, exercise programs, supplements and cutting edge research on fat-loss from around the world. www.fatwars.com <http://www. fatwars.com>, is an information network designed to give you the weapons you will need to continue on with victory after victory in the Fat Wars.

Fat Wars Daily Food Log   *Week of :*

Meal/Time	Items	Serving	Protein	Carbs	Fat	Calories
		Totals				

Comments

5: Take Responsibility for Reaching Your Goal, But Be Patient with Yourself

Don't sweat it if you lose a battle or two. None of us is perfect. Most of us, myself included, work long hours and have little time to waste. The key is to keep your eye on the big picture, which is permanent fat loss. If you slip up now and then, it won't make a big difference in the scheme of things.

Remember that changing a lifetime of bad habits—or even making minor adjustments—is not going to happen overnight. But as the story of the rock and the sand showed, if you add one grain of sand a day, eventually the rock will move. If you aren't seeing the results you are looking for in the (reasonable) time frames you have given yourself, take a hard look at your logbooks. Are you doing everything it takes to accomplish your goal? Can you take it to a new level now that you've made a start? Remember that if you take in too many calories in any form, they will be deposited in your fat account. If you rarely take your fat-burning engine out for a spin, that stored fuel is going to stay in storage. Do everything in your power to stay on track. Just think of yourself standing in front of that full-length mirror looking at your new body, and think of yourself enjoying each day with energy to spare. How will that feel?

Congratulations! You are well on your way to a new, healthier, happier, leaner you. It's time to win the Fat Wars!

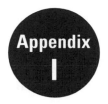

Appendix
I

Testing Testing...
Body Fat, Do You Read?

The need for an accurate measurement of percentage of body fat stems from the knowledge that the relationship of body fat to lean body mass, *not weight*, is the best measure of how lean (or not) one is. Therefore, a body mass analyzer becomes a must for health care, fitness and training professionals. This appendix describes various methods that are currently in use for determining body composition, as well as the relative advantages and disadvantages of each method.

INDIRECT METHODS

These are the methods that determine the percentage of body fat by measuring other elements, e.g., body water or thickness of skinfolds. All of these methods are based on certain assumptions.

Densitometry

Underwater weighing is the first practical method of determining body fat. In this method, there are several fundamental assumptions.

- *Assumption #1:* The human body is made up of two parts: body fat and lean muscle mass.
- *Assumption #2:* The weight of body fat is equal to 90% of equivalent water. The weight of the fat-free portion of the body is 110% of an equivalent mass of water.
- *Assumption #3:* The percentage of water in the body (level of hydration) of all people that are tested would be identical.
- *Assumption #4:* Each person would have a constant relationship in the amount of bone to muscle in the fat-free body.

It is generally accepted that underwater weighing has an accuracy within approximately 3%, with a precision of between 2 and 3%. "Accuracy" refers to the statistical relationship between the results that two separate underwater weighing facilities would calculate for the percent of body fat on the same group of individuals. "Precision," sometimes called "reproducibility" or "reliability of measurement" refers to how close the test results are when the same underwater weighing facility re-weighs the same person.

Underwater weighing requires a sophisticated water tank, in which the water is kept at a constant temperature and carefully filtered. The person is first weighed, then enters the water tank and is carefully re-weighed under water, with the head fully submerged. The tank size and subject's ability to exhale all air out of the lungs while under water affect the accuracy of the test results.

Although it is obvious that underwater weighing techniques have severe limitations, most experts use it as the "Gold Standard" and it is currently the official method of measuring body fat.

Skinfold Calipers

Using skinfold calipers is the low-cost method of measuring body fat. It is the sum of skinfold measurements at various sites of the body. There are two fundamental assumptions in developing skinfold caliper data:

- *Assumption #1:* Subcutaneous fat is equal to 50% of the total fat of the body. The assumption is more valid in younger adults than older people.
- *Assumption #2:* The various body sites selected for measurement of the skinfolds represent the average thickness of all the subcutaneous fat.

Neither of these assumptions has been proven to be true. Furthermore, the procedure depends on the judgement and skill of the person performing the measurement. Such measurements are often inaccurate—as much as three times that of underwater weighing (i.e., an accuracy within 9%).

Perhaps the biggest problem with the skinfold calipers test is the inability of even well-trained operators to produce the same measurements on the same individuals. Imprecision is why skinfold calipers are a poor method of providing meaningful information during diet programs or athletic conditioning.

Bioelectrical Impedance

This is a relatively modern method using a high-frequency, low-voltage electrical current to pass through the body. (The person tested lies down on a comfortable surface while electrodes are attached to the fingers and ankles.) This electrical current penetrates both the intra- and extra-cellular fluids and provides an accurate measurement of "body water." Therefore, if the body is assumed to be in "balance," this method allows an accurate calculation of the corresponding percentage of body fat.

The assumption that the body is in "balance" and that the body fat content is exactly related to the water content of the body requires an adherence to a strict testing protocol, which includes fasting for a considerable period of time before testing, voiding within 30 minutes of testing and avoiding physical activity for at least two hours before testing.

Provided that pre-testing protocol is met, bioelectrical impedance can provide accuracy similar to that of underwater weighing. Often, however, the pre-test protocol is not followed, so the test results may be inaccurate. Finally, bioelectrical impedance results can be quite inaccurate in pregnant or menstruating women. It cannot be used on individuals who have cardiac arythmia, especially those with cardiac pacemakers.

Other Methods

There are many other methods, such as using of radioactive tracers like detrium oxide, for determining the total amount of body water. However, all these methods are complicated, need laboratories and should be performed in a medical setting.

DIRECT METHODS

There are methods that can measure body fat content directly without calculating it from other body elements.

Near Infrared Technology (Futrex)

The technique is a method approved by the U.S. Department of Agriculture to measure the fat content of meat. It is based on the fact that near-infrared light is absorbed differently by the different organic materials constituting tissue. In other words, when such a light is shone on body tissue, body fat absorbs the light whereas lean body mass reflects the light. The reflected light is measured by a special sensor and transmitted into a computer, which has already been given data on the subject's weight, height, body frame, etc. The computer interprets all the information to produce the percentage of body fat. As the body fat is measured directly, changes in the other elements of the body (e.g., water) have no bearing on the accuracy of the measurement.

Futrex recommends measuring the body fat on a single site, the center of the biceps of the dominant arm. Independent studies show that the single-site measurement provides an accuracy within 2.8%, which is well within the range of accuracy of underwater weighing. The remarkable accuracy and ease of use have made this the most desirable method. The Futrex Website can be found at www.futrex.com.

Dual Energy X Ray Absorptometry (DEXA)

This is perhaps the most accurate way to measure body fat, lean mass and bone density. However, the procedure (the passage of X rays through the tissue) has not been approved for non-medical settings. Further, the cost of the DEXA machine (about US$60,000) is a prohibitive factor.

Extraction Method

The fat content from ground tissue is extracted and measured by a fat solvent (e.g., ether). While the method is very accurate for hamburger meat (within 0.1%), it is not practical on a human subject. (Very difficult to find volunteers!)

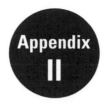

Appendix II

Fat Wars Product Supplement
Recommendations

Throughout the book there have been recommendations for supplements and other products. Below you will find some more specific suggestions. Some of these products are marketed by ehn Inc., the distributor of the award-wining greens+. I have confidently recommended these products for a number of years, believing them to be among the best in the industry. Early last year I agreed to come aboard the greens+ team and develop cutting-edge products for the company. Some of which are, transform+, proteins+, and lean+. I have no other affiliation with any other manufacturer.

Through my many years in the health industry I have come to realize there are only a handful of respectable and trustworthy product manufacturers. The recommendations I have presented here are, to the best of my knowledge, some of the top ones in the industry.

Whey Protein Isolate (proteins+ and transform+)
AlphaPure® is a patented isolation process for whey protein isolate, creating the highest biological value of any protein on the market today. AlphaPure® contains 2.5 times the cysteine levels present in other whey

protein isolates. AlphaPure® provides an excellent and unsurpassed source of natural glutathione builders.

The levels of the amino acid tryptophan in AlphaPure® are triple that of other whey protein isolates. Tryptophan is needed by the body to produce the neurotransmitter serotonin. Through extensive research over the past 40 years, it has been established that the activity level of serotonin has a material impact on levels of insomnia, pain sensitivity, anxiety and depression. Serotonin has also been demonstrated to have appetite-suppressant qualities.

AlphaPure® contains the highest levels of glycomacropeptides (GMPs) found in any whey protein product. GMPs are powerful stimulators of a hormone called cholecystokinin (CCK), which plays many essential roles in our gastrointestinal system. CCK stimulates the release of enzymes from the pancreas, and increases gallbladder contraction and bowel motility. One of CCK's most incredible actions lies in its ability to regulate our food intake by sending satiation signals to the brain, making it a potential diet aid. In animal studies, a rise in CCK is always followed by a large reduction in food intake. In human studies, whey protein glycomacropeptides were shown to increase CCK production by 415% within 20 minutes after ingestion.

AlphaPure® is distributed exclusively in Canada by ehn Inc.
ehn Inc. (Greens+ Canada)
317 Adelaide Street West, Suite 501
Toronto, Ontario, M5V 1P9
Tel: 416-977-3505
Toll-free: 877-500-7888
Fax: 416-977-4184
Web Site: www.greenspluscanada.com

AlphaPure® is a registered trademark of:
Protein Fractionations Inc.
1146 Castlefield Ave.,
Toronto, Ontario, M6B 1E9
Tel: 416-783-8315
Fax: 416-783-7589

Soy Protein Isolate

Look for the Supro® non-GMO brand of soy protein isolate. Supro® non-GMO brand of soy protein isolate contains the highest-quality water-extracted soy protein on the market today. Supro® non-GMO soy protein isolate has a biological value of 100, the same as egg, when it comes to protein quality. The product transform+ only uses Supro® non-GMO soy protein isolate as its soy protein source.

NOTE: Soy protein is a very good source of natural high tryptophan levels (stated above), as well as the muscle-building branched chain amino acids (BCAA's).

Supro® is a registered trademark of:
Protein Technologies International
P.O. Box 88940
St. Louis, Missouri, 63188
Toll-free: Consumer Inquiries: 877-SOY4HEALTH (877-769-4432)
        Customer or Business Inquiries: 800-325-7108
Fax: 314-982-2461

Essential Fatty Acid (EFA) Manufacturers and Distributors

Omega Balance Oil & Flax Oil
IN CANADA:
        Omega Nutrition Canada Inc.
        1924 Franklin Street
        Vancouver, British Columbia, V5L 1R2
        Tel: 604-253-4677
        Toll-free: 800-661-3529
        Fax: 604-253-4893
        Web Site: www.omegaflo.com
IN THE UNITED STATES:
        Omega Nutrition U.S.A. Inc.
        6515 Aldrich Road
        Bellingham, Washington 98226
        Tel: 360-384-1328
        Toll-free: 800-661-3529
        Fax: 360-384-0700
        Web Site: www.omegaflo.com

Udo's Choice Oil & Flax Oil
IN CANADA:
        Flora Distributors Ltd.
        7400 Fraser Park Drive
        Burnaby, British Columbia, V5J 5B9
        Toll-free: 800-663-0617
        Fax: 604-436-6060
        Web Site: www.florahealth.com

IN THE UNITED STATES:
Flora Distributors Ltd.
P.O. Box 73
805 Badger Road East
Lynden, Washington, 98264
Toll-free: 800-446-2110
Fax: 360-354-5355
Web Site: www.florahealth.com

Bioriginal Oils
IN CANADA:
Bioriginal Food & Science Corp.
102 Melville Street
Saskatoon, Saskatchewan, S7J 0R1
Tel: 306-975-9268
Fax: 306-242-3829

Fish Oils, EPA & DHA
IN CANADA:
Ocean Nutrition Canada Ltd.
747 Bedford Highway
Bedford, Nova Scotia, V4A 2Z7
Tel: 902-457-2399
Toll-free: 800-980-8889
Fax: 902-457-2357
Web Site: www.ocean-nutrition.com

Evening Primrose Oil (GLA)
IN CANADA:
Efamol Canada (1998) Ltd.
Scotia Centre
35 Webster Street
Kentville, Nova Scotia, B4N 1H4
Toll-free: 800-539-3326
Fax: 902-678-2885
Web Site: www.efamol.com

Flora Distributors Ltd.
7400 Fraser Park Drive
Burnaby, British Columbia, V5J 5B9
Toll-free: 800-663-0617
Fax: 604-436-6060
Web Site: www.florahealth.com

Purity Professionals (professional distributor)
Division of Purity Life Health products
2975 Lake City Way
Burnaby, British Columbia, V5A 2Z6
Toll-free: 888-443-3323
Fax: 888-223-6111
E-mail: professional@puritylife.com

Concentrated Green Foods

Not all concentrated green foods are the same quality. Look for powders that contain an array of natural organic greens and herbs. I highly recommend the multi-award-winning greens+ formula.

IN CANADA:

ehn Inc. (Greens+ Canada)
317 Adelaide Street West, Suite 501
Toronto, Ontario, M5V 1P9
Tel: 416-977-3505
Toll-free: 877-500-7888
Fax: 416-977-4184
Web Site: www.greenspluscanada.com

IN THE UNITED STATES:

Orange Peel Enterprises, Inc.
2183 Ponce de Leon Circle
Vero Beach, Florida, 32960
Toll-free: 800-643-1210
Web Site: www.greensplus.com

Green Foods Corporation
320 North Graves avenue
Oxnard, California, 93030
Tel: 805-983-7470
Toll-free: 800-777-4430
Web Site: www.greenfoods.com

Vitamins, Minerals, Antioxidants & Flavonoids

Look for formulas that contain as close a mix to the network antioxidants as possible. Vitamins C and E, Lipoic acid, and CoQ10, along with grape seed extract and a mix of the carotenoids. I am presently working on a formula for the greens+ company; however, at this time it is not ready. Look for it soon. *Full spectrum grape extract:* There are many various qualities on the market so choose wisely. Quality full spectrum grape extract formulas should contain 95% procyanidolic values with resveratrol and ellagic acid. My favorite is a product called grapes+ that contains all of the values mentioned here.

NOTE: The best way to boost glutathione levels in the body is to take lipoic acid (or Alpha Pure® protein found in proteins and transform+).

IN CANADA (coming soon, the ultimate antioxidant formula):
　　　ehn Inc. (Greens+ Canada)
　　　317 Adelaide Street West, Suite 501
　　　Toronto, Ontario, M5V 1P9
　　　Tel: 416-977-3505
　　　Toll-free: 877-500-7888
　　　Fax: 416-977-4184
　　　Web Site: www.greenspluscanada.com

Natures Secret, Natrol, Twin Lab's and other
high-quality products distributed by Purity Life:

Purity Life
6 Commerce Crescent
Acton, Ontario, L7J 2X3
Tel: 519-853-3511
Toll-free: 800-265-2615
Fax: 519-853-4660
E-mail: info@puritylife.com

Purity Professionals (distributor of
professional nutritional products)
Division of Purity Life Health products
2975 Lake City Way
Burnaby, British Columbia, V5A 2Z6
Toll-free: 888-443-3323
Fax: 888-223-6111
E-mail: professional@puritylife.com

Herbal Products & Preparations

Milk thistle: Generally, milk thistle extracts come standardized to contain a minimum of 75% silymarin. At this potency a dose of 50–100 milligrams 2–3 times daily will really boost liver cell activity and keep your fat burning army marching along toward victory. One of the most effective formulas for liver function presently on the market is called liv-tone™, marketed in Canada by:

> ehn Inc. (Greens+ Canada)
> 317 Adelaide Street West, Suite 501
> Toronto, Ontario, M5V 1P9
> Tel: 416-977-3505
> Toll-free: 877-500-7888
> Fax: 416-977-4184
> Web Site: www.greenspluscanada.com

> ***Herbal Products & Preparations recommended***
> ***in the UNITED STATES:***
>> Nature's Herbs
>> 600 East Quality Drive
>> American Fork, Utah, 84003
>> Toll-free: 1-800-437-2257
>> Fax: 801-763-0789
>> Web Site: www.twinlab.com

Carnitine

L-Carnitine is presently restricted in Canada, however it is concentrated in colostrum, and supplementing with bovine colostrum may be a great way to increase natural carnitine levels.

> *IN CANADA:*
>> Symbiotics Colostrum™, distributed by:
>> Purity Life
>> 6 Commerce Crescent
>> Acton, Ontario, L7J 2X3
>> Tel: 519-853-3511
>> Toll-free: 800-265-2615
>> Fax: 519-853-4660
>> E-mail: info@puritylife.com

>> Smarte Brand Laboratories Ltd.
>> 610F - 70 Avenue SE
>> Calgary, Alberta, T2H 2J6
>> Tel: 403-252-7150
>> Fax: 403-258-0689
>> E-mail: smarte@smarte.ab.ca

IN THE UNITED STATES:
>Symbiotics, Inc.
>2301 W Hwy 89A, Suite 107
>Sedona, Arizona, 86336
>Toll-Free: 800-784-4355
>Local phone: 520-203-0277
>Fax: 520-203-0279
>Web Site: www.symbiotics.com

Pharmaceutical Grade L-Carnitine & Acetyl L-Carnitine
ONLY IN THE UNITED STATES:
>Twin Laboratories Inc.
>2120 Smithtown Avenue
>Ronkonkoma, New York, 11779
>Tel: 631-467-3140
>Fax: 631-630-3486
>Web Site: www.twinlab.com

>Life Extension Foundation (mail order only)
>995 South West 24th Street
>Ft. Lauderdale, Florida, 33315
>Tel: 954-766-8433
>Toll-free: 800-841-5433
>Fax: 954-921-2069
>Web Site: www.lef.org

lean+: The ultimate Fat Wars nutrient formula

While there are a number of fat-burning nutrients listed individually, you don't have to hunt each of them down. Many can be found in combination with other fat-burning nutrients in a special cocktail available as lean+. Designed by author Brad King, it contains seven of the star players in the war on fat: Citrus Aurantium (Bitter Orange or Zhi Chi); Hydroxycitric Acid (HCA); Coleus Foskohlii extract; Gugulipid; Green Tea extract; Alpha Lipoic Acid and Cayenne. Many of these were introduced in Chapter 12.

lean+ is a unique formula that targets BAT cell stimulation as well as a variety of other biochemical problems inherent to weight loss, including the activation of the enzymes and messengers necessary for fat loss to occur.

lean+

- Stimulates BAT cells thus increasing the body's capacity to burn calories without exercise.
- Increases the breakdown of stored fat (lipolysis) by activating fat-releasing enzymes and increasing intracellular communication.

- Increases the metabolic rate through increased thermogenesis (body heat production) and stimulation of the thyroid.
- Curbs excess appetite.
- Improves the metabolism of carbohydrates (sugars) so less convert to fat.
- Inhibits the production of fat by the fat cells.
- Increases energy.
- Lowers LDL and VLDL ("bad") cholesterol levels while increasing HDL ("good") cholesterol levels.
- Protects against damage by free radicals.

Ingredient Highlights:
- Alpha lipoic acid—is not only a potent antioxidant that helps to protect virtually all the tissues of the body, but also is a cofactor for some of the key enzymes (alpha keto acid dehydrogenases) involved in generating energy from food and oxygen in mitochondria.
- Alpha lipoic acid—also helps to control excess sugar levels by improving carbohydrate metabolism and ensuring fewer carbohydrates (sugars) are converted into fat. This also improves energy levels as the metabolized carbohydrates become energy for your mind and body.
- Cayenne—stimulates the production of ATP (fuel), thus increasing thermogenesis and stimulating the BAT cells so more calories are burned. It also aids in the absorption of the other ingredients.
- *Citrus aurantium*—increases the breakdown of stored fat (lipolysis) by increasing the activity of the BAT cells and thus thermogenesis and the metabolic rate. Unlike ephedra (Ma huang), caffeine or guarana, *Citrus aurantium* works by attaching its amines to the Beta-3 (thermogenic receptor) receptor sites on a cell's surface without stimulating the central nervous system and thus has none of the associated side effects or health risks.
- *Coleus forskohlii*—increases the breakdown of stored fat (lipolysis) through the increase of the cellular messenger cAMP (cyclic adenosine monophosphate) in cells.
- Grapefruit juice powder—for those who remember the popular grapefruit diet of the '70s, here is the reason it worked. Grapefruit contains pectin, which helps to lower fat absorption and suppress the appetite. In lean+, the grapefruit juice powder complements the *Citrus aurantium* for increased efficacy.

- Green tea—regulates the appetite and increases the activity of BAT cells, thus increasing thermogenesis and burning excess fat and calories. Green tea may also lower fat absorption by the intestines, and inhibit excess carbohydrates from being absorbed (inactivates amylase activity).
- Guggulipid—contains plant compounds called guggulsterones that have been proven to regulate the metabolism by stimulating thyroid output by helping to convert inactive thyroid hormones into metabolically active ones (T4-T3). This in turn stimulates the BAT cells, increasing thermogenesis and burning stored fat. Guggulipid also lowers the risk of coronary artery disease and "bad" cholesterol (LDL and VLDL) levels—both commonly associated with obesity.
- Hydroxycitric acid (HCA) from *Garcinia cambogia*—curbs the appetite, inhibits the conversion of carbohydrates (sugars) into fat, reduces fat production and storage, and improves the rate of fat burning in cells by inhibiting an enzyme that blocks fat from being burnt (malonyl CoA).

IN CANADA:

> *lean+ is manufactured and distributed by:*
> ehn Inc. (Greens+ Canada)
> 317 Adelaide Street West, Suite 501
> Toronto, Ontario, M5V 1P9
> Tel: 416-977-3505
> Toll-free: 877-500-7888
> Fax: 416-977-4184
> Web Site: www.greenspluscanada.com

NOTE: Look for updated information on products, exercises and research on the *Fat Wars* web site: **www.fatwars.com**

Dr. Seaton's Advanced Hygiene System (see Chapter 2)

is available from:
High Performance Hygiene
24000 Mercantile Road, Suite 7
Cleveland, Ohio, 44122
Tel/Toll-free: 888-262-5700
Fax/Toll-free: 888-247-8500
Web Site: www.advancedhealth.cc

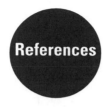

References

CHAPTER 1: THE SKINNY ON FAT—THE GENERATOR AND THE FURNACE

Astrup, A., et al. "Pharmacology of thermogenic drugs," *Am J of Clin Nutr*, 1992.

Barenys M.; Recasens M.A.; Martí Henneberg C; Salas Salvadó J. "Effect of Exercise and Protein Intake on Energy Expenditure in Adolescents," *Rev Esp Fisiol*, Dec, 1993, 49:4, 209-17.

Barnes, BO., & Galton, L.; *Hypothyroidisim: The Unsuspected Illness*. New York: Harper & Row, 1976.

Berry, M., et al., "The Contribution of Hepatic Metabolism to Diet-Induced Thermogenesis," *Metabolism*, 1985; 34: 141-147.

Brent, GA.; "The Molecular Basis of Thyroid Action," *N Engl J Med*, 1994, 331: 847-853,

Collins, S., et al. "Strain Specific Response to Beta-3 Adrenergic Receptor agonist Treatment of Diet Induced Obesity in Mice," *Endocrinol*, 1997; 138: 405-413.

Dulloo A.G., Miller D.S. "The Thermogenic Properties of Ephedrine/methylxanthine Mixtures: Human Studies," *Int J Obesity*, 1986:10: 467-481

Fleury, C., et al. "Uncoupling protein-2: A Novel Gene Linked to Obesity and Hyperinsulinemia," *Nat Genetics*, 1997, 15: 269-272.

Ghorbam, M., et al; "Hypertrophy of Brown Adipocytes in Brown and White Adipose Tissues and Reversal of Diet Induced Obesity in Rats Treated with a Beta-3 Adrenoceptor Agonist," *Biochem Pharmacol*, 1997, 54: 121-131.

Gura, T; "Uncoupling Proteins Provide New Clue to Obesity's Causes," *Science* May 29; 1998, 280: 1369-1370.

Harper M.E., Faculty of Medicine, University of Ottawa, "Obesity Research Continues to Spring Leaks," *Clin Invest Med* Aug; 20: 239-44.

James W.P.T., Trayhum P. "Thermogenesis and obesity," *British Med Bulletin*, 1981, 37(1): 43-48

Kaats, G., "Effects of Multiple Herbal Formulation on Body Composition, Blood, Chemistry, Vital Signs and Self-reported Energy Levels and Appetite Control," *Int J Obesity*, 1994.

Kopecky, J, "Mitochondrial Energy Metabolism, Uncoupling Proteins and Adipose Tissue Accumulation," *Sb Lek* 1998, 99 (3): 219-25.

Mersmann, H., "Evidence of Classic Beta 3 Adrenergic Receptors in Porcine Adipocytes," *J Anim Sci*, May, 1996, 74:5: 984-92.

Ricquier D, "Uncoupling Protein-2 (UCP2): Molecular and Genetic Studies," *Int J Obes Relat Metab Disord* Jun, 1999, 23 Suppl 6: S38-42

Salas, SJ, "Influence of Adiposity on the Thermic Effect of Food and Exercise in Lean and Obese Adolescents," *Int J Obes Relat Metab Disord*, Dec., 17, 1993, 12: 717-22.

Schrauwen P; Troost FJ; Xia J; Ravussin E; Saris WH, "Skeletal Muscle UCP2 and UCP3 Expression in Trained and Untrained Male Subjects" *Int J Obes Relat Metab Disord* Sep, 1999 (9): 966-72

Schrauwen P; Walder K; Ravussin E, "Human uncoupling proteins and obesity," *Obes Res* Jan, 1999; 7(1): 97-105

Yang, Y., et al. "Multiple Actions of Beta Adrenergic Agonists on Skeletal Muscle and Adipose Tissue," *Biochem J*, 1989.

CHAPTER 2: HORMONES, PROTEINS AND FAT BURNING

Cassidy, C.M., "Nutrition and Health in Agriculturists and Hunter-gatherers: A Case Study of Two Prehistoric Populations," *Nutritional Anthropology*, Pleasantville, New York: 117-145.

Crist D.M., et al; "Body Composition Response to Exogenous GH during Training in Highly Conditioned Adults," *J Appl Physiol*, Aug 1988, 65:2: 579-84.

Curtis, H. *Biology*, 4th ed. New York: Worth Publishers, 1986.

Dilman, V.M. *The Grand Biological Clock*. Moscow: Mir, 1989.

Eaton SB, Eaton SB III, Konner MJ, et al., "An Evolutionary Perspective Enhances Understanding of Human Nutritional Requirements," *J of Nutr*, June 1996;126: 1732-40.

Eaton, S.B., "Humans, Lipids and Evolution," *Lipids*, 1992; 27(10): 814-820.

Goldwasser P., Feldman J. "Association of Serum Albumin and Mortality Risk," *J Clin Epidemiol*, 1997, 50: 693-703.

Klatz, R. & Kahn, C. *Grow Young with HGH*. New York: HarperCollins, 1997.

Patterson C.R. *Essentials of Biochemistry*, Pittman Books, London, 1983, 38.

Peters T. *All About Albumin*, Academic Press, San Diego, 1996.

Samra J.S., et al. "Suppression of the Nocturnal Rise in Growth Hormone Reduces Subsequent Lipolysis in Subcutaneous Adipose Tissue." *Eur J Clin Invest*, 1999, 29 (12): 1045-52.

Seaton K. "Carrying Capacity of Blood in Aging." Presented at the Anti-Aging conference, Las Vegas, 1999. Abstract available from Advanced Health Products, LLC, Beachwood, Ohio. Ph: 1-888-262-5700.

Sonntag W., et al; "Moderate Caloric Restriction Alters the Subcellular Distribution of Somatostatin mRNA and Increases Growth Hormone Pulse Amplitude in Aged Animals," *Neuroendocrinology*, May, 1995, 61:5: 601-8.

Sonntag W.E., et al; "Pleiotropic Effects of Growth Hormone and Insulin-like Growth Factor (IGF)-1 on Biological Aging: Inferences from Moderate Caloric-restricted Animals," *J Gerontol A Biol Sci Med Sci*, Dec, 1999, 54:12: B521-38.

Xu X; Sonntag W.E.; "Moderate Caloric Restriction Prevents the Age-related Decline in Growth Hormone Receptor Signal Transduction," *J Gerontol A Biol Sci Med Sci*, Mar, 1996, 51:2: B167-74.

Yudkin, J., "Evolutionary and Historical Changes in Dietary Carbohydrates," *Amer J Clin Nutr*, 1967; 20(2): 108-115.

CHAPTER 3: HIS FAT

Barnhart, Edward R. *Physicians' Desk Reference*, 45th ed. Oradell, NJ: Medical Economics Co., 1991.

Bhasin, S., et al. "The Effects of Supraphysiologic Doses of Testosterone on Muscle Size and Strength in Normal Men." *New Engl J Med*, July 1996, 335, no. 1: 1–7.

BPH, "The Other Side of the Coin." *Life Extension*, February 1999.

Campbell, D.R., and M.S. Kurzer. "Flavonoid Inhibition of Aromatase Enzyme Activity in Human Preadipocytes." *J Steroid Biochem Mol Biol* Sept 1993, 46, no. 3,: 381–8.

Fisher, B., et al. "Strength Training Parameters in the Edmonton Police Force Following Supplementation with Elk Velvet Antler (EVA)." 1998.

Hryb, D.J., et al. "The Effect of Extracts of the Roots of the Stinging Nettle (*Urtica dioica*) on the Interaction of SHBG with Its Receptor on Human Prostatic Membranes." *Planta Med* 61, no. 1 (February 1995):31–2.

Hsieh, C., and J. Granstrom. "Staying Young Forever: Putting New Research Findings into Practice." *Life Extension* (December 1999).

_____, et al. "Predictors of Sex Hormone Levels Among the Elderly: A Study in Greece." *J of Clin Endocrinology and Metab* 51, no. 10, October 1999: 837–41.

Isidori, A.M., et al. "Leptin and Androgens in Male Obesity: Evidence for Leptin Contribution to Reduced Androgen Levels." *Journal of Clinical Endocrinology and Metabolism* 84, no. 10 October 1999:3673–80.

Kaplowitz, P. "Delayed Puberty in Obese Boys: Comparison with Constitutional Delayed Puberty and Response to Testosterone Therapy." *J of Pediatrics* 133, no. 6 (December 1998):745–9.

Rosmond, R., and P. Björntorp. "Endocrine and Metabolic Aberrations in Men with Abdominal Obesity in Relation to Anxio-depressive Infirmity." *Metabolism* 47, no. 10 (October 1998):1187–93.

_____, and P. Björntorp. "The Interactions between Hypothalamic-Pituitary-Adrenal Axis Activity, Testosterone, Insulin-like Growth Factor I and Abdominal Obesity with Metabolism and Blood Pressure in Men." *Int J Obes Relat Metab Disord* Dec 1998, 22, no. 12:1184–96.

Schöttner, M., et al. "Lignans from the Roots of *Urtica dioica* and their Metabolites Bind to Human Sex Hormone Binding Globulin (SHBG)." *Planta Med*, Dec 1997, 63, no. 6: 529–32.

Shippen, E., and W. Fryer. *The Testosterone Syndrome: The Critical Factor for Energy, Health and Sexuality*. New York: M. Evans and Company, 1998.

Swartz, C. "Low Serum Testosterone: A Cardiovascular Risk in Elderly Men." In *Geriatric Med Today* 7, Dec 1998, no. 12.

Tchernof, A., et al. "Relationships between Endogenous Steroid Hormone, Sex Hormone-Binding Globulin and Lipoprotein Levels in Men: Contribution of Visceral Obesity, Insulin Levels and Other Metabolic Variables." *Atherosclerosis* Sept 133, no. 2: 235–44.

Vermeulen, A., et al. "Testosterone, Body Composition and Aging." *J Endocrinol Invest*, 1999, 22, no. 5: 110–6.

Volek, J.S., et al. "Testoserone and Cortisol in Relationship to Dietary Nutrients and Resistance Exercise." *J of Applied Physiology* 82, no. 1 (January 1997):49–54.

Wright, J., and L. Lenard. *Maximize Your Vitality & Potency: For Men over 40*. Petaluma, CA: Smart Publications, 1999

CHAPTER 4: HER FAT

Backstrom, T. "Neuroendocrinology of Premenstrual Syndrome." *Clin Obset & Gynecol* 35 (1992):612.

Barnes, S. "The Chemopreventive Properties of Soy Isoflavonoids in Animal Models of Breast Cancer." *Breast Cancer Res Treat*, Nov 1997, 46:2–3, 169–79.

_____, et al. "Soy Isoflavonoids and Cancer Prevention. Underlying Biochemical and Pharmacological Issues." *Adv Exp Med Biol*, 401 (a996): 87–100.

Baumgartner, R.N., et al. "Associations of Fat and Muscle Masses with Bone Mineral in Elderly Men and Women." *Am J of Clin Nutr,* 63: 365.

Bouchard, C., et al. "Inheritance of the Amount and Distribution of Human Body Fat." *Int J Obesity,* 1988, 12: 205.

Castleman, M. *The Healing Herbs.* New York: Bantam, 1995.

Cauley, J.A., et al. "The Epidemiology of Serum Sex Hormones in Postmenopausal Women." *Am J Epidem,* 1989, 129: 1120.

Ferraro, R., et al. "Lower Sedentary Metabolic Rates in Women Compared with Men." *J Clin Invest,* 1992, 90: 780.

Futagawa, N.K., et al. "Effect of Age on Body Composition and Resting Metabolic Rate." *Am J Physiol,* 1990, 259: E233.

Ingram, D., et al. "Case-Control Study of Phytoestrogens and Breast Cancer." *Lancet,*.Oct 1997, 350: 990–94.

Kaym, S., et al. "Associations of Body Mass and Fat Distribution with Sex Hormone Concentrations in Postmenopausal Women." *Int J Epidemiol,* 1991, 151

Knudsen, C. "Super Soy: Health Benefits of Soy Protein." *Energy Times,* Feb 1996:12.

Laux, M., and C. Conrad. *Natural Woman, Natural Menopause.* New York: HarperCollins Inc., 1998.

Ley, C.J., et al. "Sex and Menopausal Associated Changes in Body Fat Distribution." *Am J of Clin Nutr,* 1992, 55: 950.

Mauriège, P., et al. "Abdominal Fat Cell Lipolysis, Body Fat Distribution, and Metabolic Variables in Premenopausal Women." *J of Clin Endocrinology and Metab,* Oct 1990.

Messina, M.J., et al. Second International Symposium on the Role of Soy in Preventing and Treating Chronic Diseases, Brussels (September 19, 1996): 36.

Mindell, E. *Earl Mindell's Soy Miracle.* New York: Simon & Schuster, 1995.

Pasquali, R., et al. "Body Weight, Fat Distribution and the Menopausal Status in Women." *Int J Obesity,* 1994, 18, no. 9: 614–21.

Rink, J.D., et al. "Cellular Characterization of Adipose Tissue from Various Body Sites of Women." *J of Clin Endocrinology and Metab,* July 1996.

Simpson, E. "Regulation of Estrogen Biosynthesis by Human Adipose Cells." *Endocrin Rev,* 1989, 10: 136.

Walker, M. "Concentrated Soybean Phytochemicals." *Healthy & Natural Journal,* 1994, 2, no. 2.

———."Phytochemicals in Soybeans." *Health Foods Business,* March 1995: 36.

Waterhouse, D. *Outsmarting the Midlife Fat Cell*. New York: Hyperion, 1998.

Zamboni, M., et al. "Body Fat Distribution in Pre and Post-menopausal Women: Metabolic and Antropometric Variables in the Interrelationships." *Int J Obesity*, 1992, 16: 495.

CHAPTER 5: BABY FAT

Bar-Or, O., et al. "Physical Activity, Genetic, and Nutritional Considerations in Childhood Weight Management." *Med Sci Sports Exerc*, 1998, 30, no. 1: 2–10.

Bellizi, M.C., and W.H.Dietz. "Workshop on Childhood Obesity: Summary of the Discussion." *Am J of Clin Nutr* (1999 supplement), 70:173S-5S.

Birch, L.L. "Development of Food Acceptance Patterns in the First Years of Life." *Proc Nutr Soc*, 1998, 57, no. 4: 617–24.

Caprio, S., et al. "Metabolic Impact of Obesity in Childhood." *Endocrinol Metab Clin North Am*, 1999, 28, no. 4: 731–47.

Cutting, T.M., et al. "Like Mother, Like Daughter: Familial Patterns of Overweight Are Mediated by Mothers' Dietary Disinhibition." *Am J of Clin Nutr*, 1999, 69, no. 4: 608–13.

Dewey, K.G., et al. "Breast-Fed Infants Are Leaner Than Formula-Fed Infants at 1 Year of Age: The DARLING Study." *Am J of Clin Nutr, Feb 1993* 57, no. 2: 140–45.

Ebbeling, C.B., and N.R. Rodriguez. "Effects of Exercise Combined with Diet Therapy on Protein Utilization in Obese Children." *Med Sci Sports Exerc*, 1999, 31, no. 3: 378–85.

Fallon, S., and M.Enig. "Tragedy and Hype, The Third International Soy Symposium." *Nexus Magazine*, Apr-May 2000, 7, no. 3.

Golan, M.I., et al. "Parents as the Exclusive Agents of Change in the Treatment of Childhood Obesity." *Am J of Clin Nutr*, 1998, 67, no. 6: 1130–35.

_____, et al. "Role of Physical Activity in the Prevention of Obesity in Children." *Int J Obes Relat Metab Disord* (Supplement 3 1999), 23: S18–33.

_____, and B.A. Gower. "Relation Between Visceral Fat and Disease Risk in Children and Adolescents." *Am J of Clin Nutr* (1999 supplement), 70: 149S–56S.

Irvine, C., et al. "The Potential Adverse Effects of Soybean Phytoestrogens in Infant Feeding." *New Zealand Med J* May 24, 1995: 318.

Keller, J.D., et al. "Infants of Diabetic Mothers with Accelerated Fetal Growth by Ultrasonography: Are They All Alike?" *Am J Obstet Gynec*, Sept 1990, 163, no. 3: 893–97.

Levy, J.R., et al. "The Effect of Prenatal Exposure to the Phytoestrogen Genestein on Sexual Differentiation in Rats." *Proc Soc Exp Biol Med* Jan 1995, 208, no. 1: 60–6.

Metzger, B.E., et al. "Amniotic Fluid Insulin Concentration as a Predictor of Obesity." *Arch Dis Child*, Oct 1990, 65, no. 10: 1050–52.

Patel, M.S., et al. "Overview of Pup in a Cup Model: Hepatic Lipogenesis in Rats Artificially Reared on a High-Carbohydrate Formula." *J Nutr* (Feb 1993 supplement), 123, no. 3: 373–77.

Proceedings of the Nutrition Society, 1992, 51: 353–65.

Robinson, T.N. "Does Television Cause Childhood Obesity?" *JAMA*, 1998, 279, no. 12: 959–60.

_____. "Reducing Children's Television Viewing to Prevent Obesity: A Randomized Controlled Trial." *JAMA*, 1999, 282, no. 16: 1561–67.

Rosenbloom, A.L., et al. "Emerging Epidemic of Type 2 Diabetes in Youth." *Diabetes Care*, 1999, 22, no. 2: 345–54.

Santti, R., et al. "Phytoestrogens: Potential Endocrine Disruptors in Males." *Toxicol Ind Health*, Jan 1998, 14: 1–2, 223–37.

Setchell, K.D., et al. "Isoflavone Content of Infant Formulas and the Metabolic Fate of These Early Phytoestrogens in Early Life." *Am J of Clin Nutr* (Dec 1998 supplement): 1453S–1461S.

Silverman, B.L., et al. "Long-Term Prospective Evaluation of Offspring of Diabetic Mothers." *Diabetes* 40 (December 1991, Supplement 2):121–25.

Slyper, A.H. "Childhood Obesity, Adipose Tissue Distribution, and the Pediatric Practitioner." *Pediatrics* 102, no. 1 (1998):E4.

Sothern, M.S., et al. "A Multidisciplinary Approach to the Treatment of Childhood Obesity." *Del Med J* 71, no. 6 (1999):255–61.

Story, M. "School-Based Approaches for Preventing and Treating Obesity." *Int J Obes Relat Metab Disord* 23 (1999 supplement): S43–51.

Strauss, R. "Childhood Obesity." *Curr Probl Pediatr*, 1999, 29, no. 1: 1–29.

Whitten, P.L., et al. "Phytoestrogen Influences on the Development of Behavior and Gonadotrophin Function." *Proc Soc Exp Biol Med*, Jan 1995, 208, no.1: 82–86.

CHAPTER 6: MACRO-FUEL ONE: CARBOHYDRATES

Baba, N.H. et al. "High Protein vs High Carbohydrate Hypoenergetic Diet for the Treatment of Obese Hyperinsulinemic Subjects." *Int J Obes Relat Metab Disord*, 1999, 23(11): 1202-6.

Clemens, L.H. et al. "The Effect of Eating Out on Quality of Diet in Premenopausal Women." *J Am Diet Assoc*, 1999, 99(4): 442-4.

Daly, J.W. et al. "Is Caffeine Addictive? The Most Widely Used
   Psychoactive Substance in the World Affects Same Parts of The Brain
   as Cocaine." *Lakartindningen*, 1998, 95 (51-52): 5878-83.
Drummond, S. et al. "A Critique of the Effects of Snacking on Body
   Weight Status." *Eur J Clin Nutr* 50(12): 779-83, 1996.
Garg, A. et al. "Effects of Varying Carbohydrate Content of Diet in
   Patients with Non-insulin-dependent Diabetes Mellitus." *JAMA*,
   1994, 271 (18): 1421-8.
Garrett, B.E. and Griffiths RR. "Physical Dependence Increases the Relative
   Reinforcing Effects of Caffeine Versus Placebo." *Psychopharmacology
   (Berl)*, 1998, 139 (3): 195-202.
Golay, A. et al. "Weight-loss with Low or High Carbohydrate Diet?" *Int J
   Obes Relat Metab Disord*, 1996, 20 (12): 1067-72.
Grant, W.B. "Low-fat, High-sugar Diet and Lipoprotein Profiles." *Am J
   Clin Nutr*, 1999, 70 (6): 1111-2.
Griffiths,R.R. et al. "Low-dose Caffeine Physical Dependence in Humans."
   J Pharmacol Exp Ther, 1990, 255 (3): 1123-32.
Harnack, L. et al. "Soft drink Consumption Among U.S. Children and
   Adolescents: Nutritional Consequences." *J Am Diet Assoc* 1999 (4):
   436-41.
Hughes, J.R. and Hale, K.L. Behavioral Effects of Caffeine and Other
   Methylxanthines on Children. *Exp Clin Psychopharmacol*, 1998, 6(1):
   87-95.
Jeppesen, J. et al. "Effects of Low-fat, High-carbohydrate Diets on Risk
   Factors for Ischemic Heart Disease in Postmenopausal Women."
   Am J Clin Nutr, 1997, 65(4): 1027-33.
Lavin, J.H. et al. "The Effect of Sucrose and Aspartame Sweetened Drinks
   on Energy Intake, Hunger, and Food Choice of Female, Moderately
   Restrained Eaters." *Int J Obes Relat Metab Disord*, 1997, 21(1): 37-42.
McCrory, M.A. et al. "Overeating in America: Association Between
   Restaurant Food Consumption and Body Fatness in Healthy Adult
   Men and Women Ages 19 to 80." *Obes Res*, 1999, 7(6): 564-71.
Miller, J.C. "Importance of Glycemic Index in Diabetes." *Am J Clin Nutr*,
   1994, 59: 747S-752S.
Reaven, G.M. "Do High Carbohydrate Diets Prevent the Development or
   Attenuate the Manifestations (Or Both) of Syndrome X? A
   Viewpoint Strongly Against." *Curr Opin Lipidol*, 1997, 8(1): 23-7.
Sidossis, L.S. et al. "Glucose plus Insulin Regulate Fat Oxidation by
   Controlling The Rate of Fatty Acid Entry into the Mitochondria."
   J Clin Invest, 1996, 98 (10: 2244-50.
Starc, T.J. et al. "Greater Dietary Intake of Simple Carbohydrate is
   Associated with Lower Concentrations of High-Density-Lipoprotein

Cholesterol in Hypercholesterolemic Children." *Am J Clin Nutr*, 1998, 67(6): 1147-54.

Strain, E.C. et al. "Caffeine Dependence Syndrome. Evidence from Case Histories and Experimental Evaluations." *JAMA*, 1994, 272(13): 1065-6.

Wolfe, B.M. and Piche, L.A. "Replacement of Carbohydrate by Protein |In a Conventional-fat Diet Reduces Cholesterol and Triglyceride Concentrations in Healthy Normolipidemic Subjects." *Clin Invest Med*, 1999, 22(4): 140-8.

CHAPTER 7: MACRO-FUEL TWO: DIETARY FAT

Barrsch, H. et al. "Dietary Polyunsaturated Fatty Acids and Cancers of the Breast and Colorectum Emerging Evidence for Their Role as Risk Modifiers." *Carcinogenesis*, 1999, 20(12): 2209-18.

Berry, E.M. "Dietary Fatty Acids In The Management of Diabetes Mellitus." *Am J Clin Nut*, 1997, 66 (4 Suppl): 991S-997S.

Bonnefont, J.P. et al. "Carnitine Palmitoyltransferase Deficiencies." *Mol Genet Metab*, 1999, 68(4): 424-40.

Borkman, M. et al. "The Relationship Between Insulin Sensitivity and the Fatty-Acid Composition of Skeletal-Muscle Phospholipids." *N Engl J Med* 328(4): 238-44, 1993.

Broadhurst, C.L. "Balanced Intakes of Natural Triglycerides for Optimum Nutrition: An Evolutionary and Phytochemical Perspective." *Med Hypotheses*, 1997, 49(3): 247-61.

Cesano, A et al. "Opposite Effects Of Linoleic Acid and Conjugated Linoleic Acid on Human Prostatic Cancer In SCID Mice." *Anticancer Res* 18 (3A): 1429-34, 1998.

Decsi, T. et al. "Long-chain Polyunsaturated Fatty Acids in Plasma Lipids of Obese Children." I 31(3): 305-11, 1996.

Demmelmair, H. et al. "Trans Fatty Acid Contents in Spreads and Cold Cuts Usually Consumed by Children." *Z Ernahrungswiss*, 1996, 35(3): 235-40.

Dreon, D.M. et al. "A Very Low-Fat Diet is not Associated with Improved Lipoprotein Profiles in Men With A Predominance of Large, Low-density Lipoproteins." *Am J Clin Nutr*, 1999, 69 (3): 411-8.

Garg, A. "High-monounsaturated-Fat Diets for Patients with Diabetes Mellitus: A Meta-analysis." *Am J Clin Nutr*, 1998, 67(3 Suppl): 577S-582S.

Harris, W.S. et al. "Influence of n-3 Fatty Acid Supplementation on the Endogenous Activities of Plasma Lipase." *Am J Clin Nutr* 1997, 66 (2): 254-60.

Horrocks, L.A. and Yeo, Y.K. "Health Benefits of Docosahexaenoic Acid (DHA)." *Pharmacol Res*, 1999, 40 (3): 211-25.

Ip, C. "Review of the Effects of Trans Fatty Acids, Oleic Acid, N-3 Polyunsaturated Fatty Acids, and Conjugated Linoleic Acid on Mammary Carcinogenesis in Animals." *Am J Clin Nutr*, 1997, 66 (6 Suppl): 1523S-1529S.

Kwiterovich, P.O. Jr. "The Effect Of Dietary Fat, Antioxidants, and Pro-Oxidants on Blood Lipids, Lipoproteins, and Atherosclerosis." *J Am Diet Assoc*, 1997 (7 Suppl): S31-41.

Lardinois, C.K. "The Role of Omega-3 Fatty Acids on Insulin Secretion and Insulin Sensitivity." *Med Hypotheses*, 1987, 24 (3): 243-8.

Louheranta, A.M. et al. "A High-Trans Fatty Acid Diet and Insulin Sensitivity in Young Healthy Women." *Metabolism*, 1999, 48 (7): 870-5.

Madsen, L. et al. "Eicosapentaenoic and Docosahexaenoic Acid Affect Mitochondrial and Peroxisomal Fatty Acid Oxidation in Relation to Substrate Preference." *Lipids*, 1999, 34 (9): 951-63.

Mori, T.A. et al. "Dietary Fish as a Major Component of a Weight-Loss Diet: Effect On Serum Lipids, Glucose, and Insulin Metabolism in Overweight Hypertensive Subjects." *Am J Clin Nutr*, 1999 70(5): 817-25.

Nelson, G.J.; Schmidt, P.C.; and Kelly, D.S. "Low-fat Diets Do Not Lower Plasma Cholesterol Levels in Healthy Men Compared to High-Fat Diets With Similar Fatty Acid Composition at Constant Calorie Intake" *Lipids*, 1995, 30(11): 969-76.

Phinney, S.D. "Arachadonic Acid Maldistribution in Obesity." *Lipids*, 1996, 31 Suppl: S271-4.

Phinney, S.D. "Metabolism of Exogenous and Endogenous Arachidonic Acid in Cancer." *Adv Exp Med Biol*, 1996, 399: 87-94.

Rieger, M.A. et al. "A Diet High in Fat and Meat But Low in Dietary Fibre Increases the Genotoxic Potential of Ofecal Water1". *Carcinogenesis* 1999, 20 (12): 2311-6.

Rustan, A.C. et al. "Omega-3 and Omega-6 Fatty Acids in the Insulin Resistance Syndrome." *Ann N Y Acad Sci*, 1997, 20 (827): 310-26.

Schmidt, M.A.; *Smart Fats*, North Atlantic Books, Berkeley, Cal., 1997.

Sears, B.; *The Anti-Aging Zone*, HarperCollins, Inc., New York, NY., 1999.

Simoneau, J.A. et al. "Markers of Capacity To Utilize Fatty Acids in Human Skeletal Muscle: Relation to Insulin Resistance and Obesity and Effects of Weight Loss." *FASEB J*, 1999, 13(14): 2051-60.

Simopoulos, A.P. "Is Insulin Resistance Influenced by Dietary Linoleic Acid and Trans Fatty Acids?" *Free Radic Biol Med*, 1994, 17(4): 367-72.

Tutelian, V.A. et al. "Effects of Polyunsaturated Fatty Acids of the Omega-3 Family in the Anti-Atherosclerotic Diet on the Activity of Lysosomal Lipolytic Enzymes, Mononuclear Cells and Blood Platelets of Patients with Ischemic Heart Disease." *Vopr Pitan*, 1993, (5): 17-2.

Willett, W.C. et al. "Is Dietary Fat a Major Determinant of Body Fat?" *Am J Clin Nutr*, 1998, 67: 556S-562S.

Willumsen, N. et al. "Eicosapentaenoic Acid, But Not Docosahexaenoic Acid, Increases Mitochondrial Fatty Acid Oxidation and Upregulates 2,4-Dienoyl-Coa Reductase Gene Expression in Rats." *Lipids*, 1996, 31(6): 579-92.

CHAPTER 8: MACRO-FUEL THREE: DIETARY PROTEIN

Barenys, M. et al. "Effect of Exercise and Protein Intake on Energy Expenditure in Adolescents." *Rev Esp Fisiol*, 1993, 49(4): 209-17.

Biolo, G., et al.; "An Abundant Supply of Amino-Acids Enhances the Metabolic Effect of Exercise on Muscle Protein," *Amer J Phys*, 1997, 273: E122-E129.

Bounous, G., et al; "The Influence of Dietary Whey Protein on Tissue Glutathione and the Diseases of Aging." *Clin Invest Med*, Dec 1989, 12: 6, 343-9.

Bounous, G; Gold P; "The Biological Activity of Undenatured Dietary Whey Proteins: Role of Glutathione," *Clin Invest Med*, Aug 1991, 14: 4, 296-309

Bounous, G., et al; "Evolutionary Traits in Human Milk Proteins," *Med Hypotheses*, Oct 1998, 27: 2, 133-40.

Bounous, G., et al; "The Immunoenhancing Property of Dietary Whey Protein Concentrate," *Clin Invest Med*, Aug 1988, 11: 4, 271-8

Bounous, G.; Batist G; Gold P; "Whey Proteins in Cancer Prevention." *Cancer Lett*, May 1999, 57: 2, 91-4.

Campbell, W.W. et al. "Effects of an Omnivorous Diet Compared With a Lactoovovegetarian Diet On Resistance-training-induced Changes in Body Composition and Skeletal Muscle in Older Men." *Am J Clin Nutr*, 1999, 70: 1032-9.

Chaitow, L.; *Amino Acids in Therapy*, Thorsons Publishers Inc., Rochester, VT, 1985.

Conley, E., *America Exhausted*, Vitality Press Inc, Flint, MI, 1998.

Coyne, L.L.; *Fat Won't Make You Fat*, Fish Creek Publishing, Alberta, Canada, 1998.

Demonty, I. et al. "Dietary Proteins Modulate the Effects of Fish Oil on Triglycerides in the Rat." *Lipids*, 1998, 33(9): 913-21.

Froyland, L. et al. "Mitochondrion is the Principal Target for Nutritional and Pharmacological Control of Triglyceride Metabolism." *J Lipid Res*, 1997, 38 (9): 1851-8.

Heine, W., et al. "Alpha-Lactalbumin-enriched Low-protein Infant Formulas: A Comparison to Breast Milk Feeding." *Acta Paediatr*, 1996, Sept, 85 (9): 1024-8.

Knudsen, C., *Super Soy: Health Benefits of Soy Protein*, Energy Times, Feb, 1996: 12.

Lemon, P.W. et al. "Moderate Physical Activity Can Increase Dietary Protein Needs." *Can J Appl Physiol*, 1997, 22 (5): 494-503.

McCarty, M.F. "Vegan Proteins May Reduce Risk Of Cancer, Obesity, and Cardiovascular Disease by Promoting Increased Glucagon Activity." *Med Hypotheses*, 1999, 53 (6): 459-85.

Mindell, E., *Earl Mindell's Soy Miracle*, Simon & Schuster, 1995.

Morr, C.V., Ha, E.Y. "Whey Protein Concentrates and Isolates: Processing And Functional Properties," *Crit Rev Food Sci Nutr*, 1993, 33: 6, 431-76.

Rankin, JW. "Role of Protein in Exercise." *Clin Sports Med* 18(3): 499-511, 1999.

Recommended Dietary Allowances, 10th ed., Washington DC: National Academy Press, 1989: 71.

Robinson, S.M. et al. "Protein Turnover and Thermogenesis in Response To High-Protein and High-Carbohydrate Feeding in Men." *Am J Clin Nutr*, 1990, 52 (1): 72-80.

Satterlee, L.D., et al.; "In Vitro Assay for Predicting Protein Efficiency Ratio as Measured by Rat Bioassay: Collaborative Study." *J Assoc Off Anal Chem*, Jul 1982, 65: 4, 798-809

Soucy, J. and Leblanc, J. "Protein Meals and Postprandial Thermogenesis." *Physiol Behav*, 1999, 65 (4-5): 705-.

Stroescu, V., et al.; "Effects of Supro Brand Isolated Soy Protein Supplement in Male and Female Elite Rowers." *XXVth FIMS World Congress of Sports Medicine*, Athens, Greece, 1994.

Vandewater, K. and Vickers, Z. "Higher-protein Foods Produce Greater Sensory-Specific Satiety." *Physiol Behav*, 1996, 59(3): 579-83.

Walker, M., "Concentrated soybean phytochemicals," *Healthy & Natural Journal*, 1994; Vol.2, No.2.

Walker, M., "Phytochemicals in Soybeans," *Health Foods Business*, March 1995: 36.

Westerterp, K.R. et al. "Diet Induced Thermogenesis Measured over 24h in a Respiration Chamber: Effect of Diet Composition." *Int J Obes Relat Metab Disord*, 1999, 23 (3): 287-92.

Whitehead, J.M. et al. "The Effect of Protein Intake on 24-Hour Energy Expenditure During Energy Restriction." *Int J Obes Relat Metab Disord*, 1996, 20(8): 727-32.

Wurtman, J.J., and Suffers, S.; *The Serotonin Solution*, Ballantine Books, 1997.

Zed, C and James, WP. "Dietary Thermogenesis in Obesity. Response to Carbohydrate and Protein Meals: The Effect of Beta-Adrenergic Blockage and Semi-starvation." *Int J Obes* 10 (5): 391-405, 1986.

CHAPTER 9: CONSTANT CRAVING

Birdsall, T.C. "Hydroxytryptophan: A Clinically-Effective Serotonin Precursor." *Altern Med Rev*, Aug 1998, 3, no. 4: 271–80.

Bolla, K.I., et al. "Memory Impairment in Abstinent MDMA ("Ecstasy") Users." *Neurology*, Dec 1998, 51, no. 6: 1532–37.

Dye, L., and J.E. Blundell. "Menstrual Cycle and Appetite Control: Implications for Weight Regulation." *Hum Reprod*, June 1997, 12, no. 6: 1142–51.

Heine, W., et al. "Alpha-Lactalbumin-Enriched Low-Protein Infant Formulas: A Comparison to Breast Milk Feeding." *Acta Paediatr*, Sept 1996, 85, no. 9: 1024–28.

Knudsen, C. "Super Soy: Health Benefits of Soy Protein." *Energy Times*, Feb 1996: 12.

Leibowitz, S., and T. Kim. "Impact of a Galanin Antagonist on Exogenous Galanin and Natural Patterns of Fat Ingestion." *Brain Research*, 1992, 599: 148–52.

Mindell, E. *Earl Mindell's Soy Miracle*. New York: Simon & Schuster, 1995.

Morr, C.V., and E.Y. Ha. "Whey Protein Concentrates and Isolates: Processing and Functional Properties." *Crit Rev Fod Sci Nutr*, 1993, 33, no. 6: 431–76.

Prasad, C. "Food, Mood and Health: A Neurobiologic Outlook." *Braz J Med Biol Res*, Dec 1998, 31, no. 12: 1517–27.

Toornvliet, A.C., et al. "Serotoninergic Drug-Induced Weight Loss in Carbohydrate Craving Obese Patients." *Int J Obes Relat Meb Disord*, Oct 1996, 20, no. 10: 917–20.

Wurtman, J.J. "Carbohydrate Craving: Relationship Between Carbohydrate Intake and Disorders of Mood." *Drugs* 39 (Supplement 3, 1990): 49–52.

Wurtman, J.J., and S. Suffers. *The Serotonin Solution*. New York: Ballantine Books, 1997.

Wurtman, R.J., et al. "Brain Serotonin, Carbohydrate-Craving, Obesity and Depression." *Adv Exp Med Biol* 398, 1996: 35–41.

CHAPTER 10: STARVING

Carlton, A., Lillios, I., *J Amer Diet Assoc*, 1986; 86:367-68.

Colgan, M., *Optimum Sports Nutrition*, New York, NY; Advanced Research Press, 1993.

Colgan, M., *The New Nutrition : Medicine For The Millennium*, Apple Publishing, 1995; 153-54.

Colmers, W., Cowley, M., et al. "Integration of NPY, AGRP, and Melanocortin Signals in the Hypothalamic Paraventricular Nucleus: Evidence of a Cellular Basis for the Adipostat," *Neuron*, 1999 24: 155–163.

Conley, E., *America Exhausted*, Vitality Press, Michigan, 1998.

Germano, C., Advantra Z™ : *The Natural Way to Lose Weight Safely*, Kensington Publishing Corp., 1998.

Klein S., "The War Against Obesity: Attacking a New Front," *American Journal of Clinical Nutrition*, June 1999, 69(6): 1061-1063.

Lowenstein, N.J., "Effect Of Hydroxy-Citrate on Fatty Acid Synthesis by Rat Liver in Vivo," *J Biol Chem*, 1971; 246:629-632.

Markert, D., *The Turbo-Protein diet*, BioMed International, 1999.

McGarry, J.D., et al; "Role of Carnitine in Hepatic Ketogenesis," *Proc Natl Acad Sci*, 1995; 72: 4385-4388.

McGarry, J.D., Foster, D.W., "Regulation of Hepatic Fatty Acid Production and Ketone Body Production," *Ann Rev Biochem*, 1980; 49: 395-420.

Next Nutrition, The IsoCaloric "No Diet" Fat Burning Handbook, Next Nutrition, Inc., 1996.

Rosenfeld, RD., et al., "Biochemical, biophysical, and pharmacological characterization of bacterially expressed human agouti-related protein," *Biochemistry*, Nov 1998, 37: 46, 16041-52.

Sapolsky, R., *Why Zebras Don't Get Ulcers*, W. H. Freeman and Company, New York, 1998.

Simopoulos, A., *Nutr Rev*, 1985; 43:33-40.

US News and World Report, 3 Feb., 1992.

CHAPTER 11: THE *FAT WARS* EATING PRINCIPLES

Ahlborg, G, Felig, P.; "Influence of Glucose Ingestion on Fuel-Hormone Response During Prolonged Exercise," *J Appl Physiol*, 1976;41: 683.

Biolo, G., et al; "An Abundant Supply of Amino Acids Enhances the Metabolic Effect of Exercise on Muscle Protein," *Amer J Physiol*, 1997, 273: E122-E129.

Blom, P.C.S., et al; "Effect of Different Post-Exercise Sugar Diets on the Rate Of Muscle Glycogen Synthesis," *Med & Sci in Sports & Exercise*, 1987, 19: 491-496.

Burke, E.R.; *Optimal Muscle Recovery*, Avery Publishing Group, New York, 1999.

Noakes, T.D., et al; "The Metabolic Response to Squash Including the Influence of Pre-Exercise Carbohydrate Ingestion," *S Afr Med J*, Nov. 1982, 62:20, 721-3.

CHAPTER 12: TOP TEN SUPPLEMENTS FOR FAT LOSS

Supplement #1, Protein Isolate

Bounous, G., and P. Gold. "The Biological Activity of Undenatured Dietary Whey Proteins: Role of Glutathione." *Clin Invest Med*, Aug 1991, 14: 296–309.

Knudsen, C. "Super Soy: Health Benefits of Soy Protein." *Energy Times*, Feb 1996: 12.

The Life Extension Foundation. *The Wonders of Whey Restoring Youthful Anabolic Metabolism at the Cellular Level*, May 1999.

Mindell, E. *Earl Mindell's Soy Miracle*. New York: Simon & Schuster, 1995.

Renner, E. *Milk and Dairy Products in Human Nutrition*. Munich, 1983.

Volpi, E., et al. "Exogenous Amino Acides Stimulate Net Muscle Protein Synthesis in the Elderly." *Clin Invest*, 1998, 101: 2000–07.

Walker, M. "Concentrated Soybean Phytochemicals." *Healthy & Natural Journal* 2, no. 2 (1994)

_____. "Phytochemicals in Soybeans, Health." *Foods Business*, March 1995: 36.

Supplement #2, EFAs

Harris, W.S., et al. "Influence of n-3 Fatty Acid Supplementation on the Endogenous Activities of Plasma Lipase." *American Journal of Clinical Nutrition*, 1997, 66, no. 2: 254–60.

Madsen, L., et al. "Eicosapentaenoic and Docosahexaenoic Acid Affect Mitochondrial and Peroxisomal Fatty Acid Oxidation in Relation to Substrate Preference." *Lipids*, 1999, 34, no. 9: 951–63.

Schmidt, M.A. *Smart Fats*. Berkeley: North Atlantic Books, 1997.

Simoneau, J.A., et al. "Markers of Capacity to Utilize Fatty Acids in Human Skeletal Muscle: Relation to Insulin Resistance and Obesity and Effects of Weight Loss." *FASEB J*, 1999, 13, no. 14: 2051–60.

Willett, W.C., et al. "Is Dietary Fat a Major Determinant of Body Fat?" *American Journal of Clinical Nutrition* 1998, 67: 556S–562S.

Supplement #3, Green Food Concentrate

Colgan, M., and L. Colgan. *The Flavonoid Revolution*. Vancouver: Apple Publishing, 1997.

Graci, S. *The Power of Superfoods: 30 Days That Will Change Your Life*. Toronto: Prentice Hall Canada Inc., 1997.

Supplement #4, Antioxidants

Bounous, G., and P. Gold. "The Biological Activity of Undenatured
    Dietary Whey Proteins: Role of Glutathione." *Clin Invest Med* .
    Aug 1991, 14, no. 4: 296–309.

Colgan, M. *Antioxidants: The Real Story.* Vancouver: Apple Publishing,
    1998.

Conley, E.J. *America Exhausted: Breakthrough Treatments of Fatigue and
    Fibromyalgia.* : Vitality Press Inc., 1997.

Gy, J.Y., et al. "Effects of Sesamin and Alpha-tocopherol, Individually or
    in Combination on the Polyunsaturated Fatty Acid Metabolism,
    Chemical Mediator Production, and Immunoglobulin in Sprague-
    Dawley Rats." *Biosci Biotechnol Biochem,* 1995, 59, no. 12: 2198–202.

Kagan, T., et al. "Coenzyme Q10 Can in Some Circumstances Block
    Apoptosis, and This Effect Is Mediated Through Mitochondria."
    Ann NY Acad Sci 887 (1999):31–47.

Kishi, Y., et al. "Alpha-lipoic Acid: Effect on Glucose Uptake, Sorbitol
    Pathway, and Energy Metabolism in Experimental Diabetic
    Neuropathy." *Diabetes* 1999, 48, no. 10: 2045–51.

Krinsky, N.I., et al. "Antioxidant Vitamins and Beta-carotene in Disease
    Prevention." *American Journal of Clinical Nutrition* 1995, 6, S:
    1299S–1540S.

Lang, I., et al. "Effect of the Natural Bioflavonoid Antioxidant Silymarin
    on Superoxide Dismutase (SOD) Activity and Expression in Vitro."
    Biotechnol Ther 1993, 4: 263–70.

Pressman, A.H. *Glutathione: The Ultimate Antioxidant.* The Philip Lief
    Group Inc., 1997.

Sinatra, S.T. *The Coenzyme Q10 Phenomenon.* New Canaan, CT: Keats
    Publishing, 1998.

Streeper, R.S., et al. "Differential Effects of Lipoic Acid Stereoisomers on
    Glucose Metabolism in Insulin-Resistant Skeletal Muscle." *Am J
    Physiol,* 1997, 273 (1 Pt 1): E185–91.

Supplement #5, Chromium

Grant, K.E., et al. "Chromium and Exercise Training: Effect on Obese
    Women." *Med Sci Sports Exerc,* 1997, 29, no. 8: 992–98.

Kaats, G.R., et al. "A Randomized, Double-Masked, Placebo-Controlled
    Study of the Effects of Chromium Picolinate Supplementation on
    Body Composition: A Replication and Extension of a Previous
    Study." *Curr Ther Res* 1998, 59: 379–88.

Vincent, J.B. "Mechanisms of Chromium Action: Low-Molecular-Weight
    Chromium-Binding Substance." *J Am Coll Nutr* 1999, 18, no. 1:
    6–12.

Supplement #6, Citrus aurantium

Astrup, A., et al. "Pharmacology of Thermogenic Drugs." *American Journal of Clinical Nutrition*, 1992.

Berry, M., et al. "The Contribution of Hepatic Metabolism to Diet-Induced Thermogenesis." *Metabolism* 1985, 34: 141–47.

Collins, S., et al. "Strain Specific Response to Beta-3 Adrenergic Receptor Agonist Treatment of Diet Induced Obesity in Mice." *Endocrinol*, 1997, 138: 405–13.

Fleury, C., et al. "Uncoupling Protein-2: A Novel Gene Linked to Obesity and Hyperinsulinemia." *Nat Genetics*, 1997, 15: 269–72.

Gurley, B.J., et al. "Ephedrine Pharmacokinetics After the Ingestion of Nutritional Supplements Containing Ephedra Since (Ma Huang)." *Ther Drug Monit* 20, no. 4 (1998):439–45.

Kaats, G. "Effects of Multiple Herbal Formulation on Body Composition, Blood, Chemistry, Vital Signs and Self-Reported Energy Levels and Appetite Control." *Int J Obesity* (1994)

Mersmann, H. "Evidence of Classic Beta-3 Adrenergic Receptors in Porcine Adipocytes." *J Anim Sci*, May 1996, 74, no. 5: 984–92.

Yang, Y., et al. "Multiple Actions of Beta Adrenergic Agonists on Skeletal Muscle and Adipose Tissue." *Biochem J* (1989)

Supplement #7, Hydroxycitric Acid

Lowenstein, N. "Effect of Hydroxycitrate on Fatty Acid Synthesis by Rat Liver in vitro." *J Biol Chem* (1971)

McGarry, J., and D. Foster. "Regulation of Hepatic Fatty Acid Production and Ketone Body Production." *Ann Rev Biochem* (1980)

Novin, D., et al. *American Journal of Clinical Nutrition* 1985, 42: 1050–62.

Sullivan, A., *American Journal of Clinical Nutrition* 30 (1977):767–76.

Supplement #8, Forskolin

Ahmad, F., et al. "Insulin and Glucagon Releasing Activity of Coleonol (Forskolin) and Its Effects on Blood Glucose Level in Normal and Alloxan Diabetic Rats." *Acta Diabetol Lat*, Jan 1991, 28, no. 1: 71–77.

Metzger, H., and E. Lindner. "The Positive Inotropic-Acting Forskolin, a Potent Adenylate Cyclase Activator." *Arzneimittelforschung* 1981, 31, no. 8: 1248–50.

Murray, M. "The Unique Pharmacology of *Coleus Forskohlii*." *Health Counselor* 7, no. 2

Seamon, K. "Structure-Activity Relationships for Activation of Adenylate Cyclase by the Diterpene Forskolin and Its Derivatives." *J Med Chem*, March 1983, 26, no. 3: 436–39.

Supplement #9, Green Tea Extract

Deng, Z., et al. "Effect of Green Tea and Black Tea on Blood Glucose, Triglycerides, and Antioxidants in Aged Rats." *J Agricult Food Chem* 1998, 46: 3875–78.

Dulloo, A. "Efficacy of a Green Tea Extract Rich in Catechin Polyphenols and Caffeine in Increasing 24h. Energy Expenditure and Fat Oxidation in Humans." *American Journal of Clinical Nutrition* 1999, 70: 1040–45.

Hara, Y. "Influence of Tea Catechins on the Digestive Tract." *J Cel Biochem*

Kreydiyyeh, S., et al. "Tea Extract Inhibits Absorption of Glucose and Sodium in Rats." *Comp Biochem Physiol C Pharmacol Toxicol Endocrinol,* 1994, 108: 359–65.

Yokogoshi, H., et al. "Effect of Theanine, R-Glutamylethylamide, on Brain Monoamines and Striatal Dopamine Release in Conscious Rats." *Neurochem Res* 1998, 46: 2143–50.

Supplement #10, Carnitine

Clouet, P., et al. "Effect of Short- and Long-Term Treatments by a Low Level Dietary L-carnitine on Parameters Related to Fatty Acid Oxidation in Winstar Rat." *Biochem Biophys Acta* 1996, 1299, no. 2: 191–97.

McGarry, J.D. "More Direct Evidence for a Malonyl-CoA-Carnitine Palmitoyltransferase I Interaction as a Key Event in Pancreatic Beta-Cell Signaling." *Diabetes,* 1994, 43: 878–83.

Paulson, D.J. "Carnitine Deficiency-Induced Cardiomyopathy." *Mol Cell Biochem,* 1998, 180: 33–41.

Reyes, B., et al. "Effects of L-carnitine on Erythrocyte Acyl-CoA, Free CoA, and Glycerophospholipid Acyltransferase in Uremia." *American Journal of Clinical Nutrition* 1998, 67, no. 3: 386–90.

Rubaltelli, F.F., et al. "Carnitine & the Premature Biol Neonate."

CHAPTER 13: GETTING PHYSICAL

Andrews, J.F. "Exercise for Slimming." *Proc Nutr Soc* Aug 1991, 50, no. 2: 459–71.

Brynr, R.W., et al. "Effects of Resistance vs. Aerobic Training Combined with an 800 Calorie Liquid Diet on Lean Body Mass and Resting Metabolic Rate." *J Am Coll Nutr,* 1999, 18, no. 2: 115–21.

Borsheim, E., et al. "Adrenergic Control of Post-exercise Metabolism." *Acta Physiol Scand,* March 1998, 162, no. 3: 313–23.

Burke, E.R. *Optimal Muscle Recovery.* New York: Avery Publishing Group, 1999.

Carlson, L.A., et al. "Studies on Blood Lipids During Exercise." *J Lab Clin Med* 1963, 61: 724–29.

Chilibeck, P.D., et al. "Higher Mitochondrial Fatty Acid Oxidation Following Intermittent Versus Continuous Endurance Exercise Training." *Can J Physiol Pharmacol*, Sept 1998, 76, no. 9: 891–94.

Coggan, A.R., et al. "Fat Metabolism During High-Intensity Exercise in Endurance-Trained and Untrained Men." *Metabolism*, 2000, 49, no. 1: 122–28.

Colgan, M. *The New Nutrition*, Chapter 25. Vancouver: Apple Publishing, 1995.

Fernández, Pastor V.J., et al. "Function of Growth Hormone in the Human Energy Continuum During Physical Exertion." *Rev Esp Fisiol, Dec 1991*, 47, no. 4: 223–29.

Herring, J.L., et al. "Effect of Suspending Exercise Training on Resting Metabolic Rate in Women." *Med Sci Sports Exerc* Jan 1992, 24, no. 1: 59–65.

Hunter, G.R., et al. "A Role for High-Intensity Exercise on Energy Balance and Weight Control." *Int J Obes Relat Metab Disord*, 1998, 22, no. 6: 489–93.

Kraemer, W.J., et al. "Effects of Heavy-Resistance Training on Hormonal Response Patterns in Younger and Older Men." *J Appl Physiol* 1999, 87, no. 3: 982–92.

McCartney, N.A., et al. "Usefulness of Weightlifting Training in Improving Strength and Maximal Power Output in Coronary Artery Disease." *Amer J Cardiol*, 1991, 67: 939.

Pavlou, K.N., et al. "Effects of Dieting and Exercise on Lean Body Mass, Oxygen Uptake and Strength." *Med Sci Sports Exer*, 1985, 17: 466–71.

Poehlman, E.T. "A Review: Exercise and Its Influence on Resting Energy Metabolism in Man." *Med Sci Sports Exerc*, Oct 1989, 21, no. 5: 515–25.

Sears, B. *The Anti-Aging Zone*. New York: Regan Books, 1999.

van Dale, D., et al. "Weight Maintenance and Resting Metabolic Rate 18–40 Months After a Diet/Exercise Treatment." *Int J Obes* April 1990, 14, no. 4: 347–59.

CHAPTER 14: *FAT WARS* ACTION PLAN

Batmanghelidj, F. *Your Body's Many Cries for Water*. Falls Church, VA: Global Health Solutions, 1998.

Burke, E.R. *Optimal Muscle Recovery*. Garden City Park, NY: Avery Publishing Group, 1999.

Fleck, S.J., and W.J. Kraemer. *Periodization Breakthrough*. New York: Advanced Research Press, 1996.

Index